Weights
on the Ball
Workbook

W9-AAC-660

Weights
on the Ball
Ball
Workbook

**Step-by-step guide
with over 350 photos**

STEVEN STIEFEL

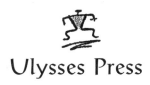

Ulysses Press

Published in the United States by Ulysses Press
P.O. Box 3440
Berkeley, CA 94703
www.ulyssespress.com

ISBN10: 1-56975-412-8
ISBN13: 978-1-56975-412-2
Library of Congress Control Number 2004101026

Printed in Canada by Webcom

10 9 8 7 6 5 4 3

Editorial/Production	Lily Chou, Claire Chun, Steven Zah Schwartz
	James Meetze
Design	Sarah Levin
Photography	Robert Holmes
Models	Andrea Alejandro, Laura Copenhaver, David Reid, Steven Stiefel

Distributed by Publishers Group West

Please Note
This book has been written and published strictly for informational purposes, and in no way
should be used as a substitute for consultation with health care professionals. You should not
consider educational material herein to be the practice of medicine or to replace consultation
with a physician or other medical practitioner. The author and publisher are providing you
with information in this work so that you can have the knowledge and can choose, at your
own risk, to act on that knowledge. The author and publisher also urge all readers to be
aware of their health status and to consult health care professionals before beginning any
health program.

ACKNOWLEDGEMENTS

This book has been a true collaboration from the outset and, first and foremost, I'd like to
thank all the great people at Ulysses Press—Lynette for seeking me out and pitching the
project to me in the first place, Bryce for all his insight and guidance, and Lily for all her
hard work and diligence, as well as all the others who spent hours on the book.

I'd like to thank all the models, especially David and Andrea, who allowed me to experiment on them with these programs as the book took shape. All three—David, Laura and
Andrea—are true professionals, and the photo shoot would not have been successful without
them. And a heartfelt thanks to Robert Holmes for his excellent photography and patience.

Finally, I'd like to thank all the people at Weider Publications who helped me with this
project, particularly: Jim Stoppani, Ph.D., for his technical edits; Mario Pacifici for his market-
ing acumen; and Anne Russell, Editor-in-Chief of *Shape Magazine*, for her insights about the
publishing world.

contents

INTRODUCTION   2
The Benefits of "Weight"-ing   3
Add a Little Balance to Your Life   5
Muscle Matters   6
Equipped for Success   8
Form and Effort   11
Warming Up and Stretching   13
Cardio Concerns   15

PART TWO: PROGRAMMED FOR SUCCESS
Let's Get Personal: An Overview   18
Firm Foundation   20
    Level 1   22
    Level 2   24
    Level 3   26
Slim and Trim   28
    Level 1   30
    Level 2   32
    Level 3   34
Muscle Bound   36
    Level 1   38
    Level 2   40
    Level 3   42

PART THREE: THE EXERCISES
Weights on the Ball: Time for Action   47
Seat of Power: Seated on the Ball   49
    Alternate Biceps Curls 50
    Hammer Curls   52
    Triceps Extensions   54
    Triceps Kickbacks   56
    Lateral Raises   58
    Shoulder Presses   60
    Front Raises   62
    Shrugs   64
Back to Basics: Back on the Ball   67
    Flat Chest Presses   68
    Incline Chest Presses   70
    Flat Chest Flyes   72
    Incline Chest Flyes   74
    Pullovers   76
    Triceps Extensions   78
    Incline Curls   80
Keeping Up a Good Front: Chest on the Ball   83
    Rear Delt Flyes   84
    Front Raises   86

Shoulder Rotations   88
Preacher Curls   90
Wrist Curls (Palm Up)   92
Wrist Curls (Palm Down)   93
Planges   94
Dumbbell Rows   96
Give Yourself a Hand: Hands on the Ball   99
    Push-ups   100
    Triceps Kickbacks   102
    Dumbbell Rows   104
    Walk-arounds   106
Amazing Feet of Strength: Feet on the Ball   109
    Push-ups   110
    Pike Presses   112
    Walk-arounds   114
    Triceps Dips   116
Get a Leg Up: Leg Strengtheners   119
    Back Extensions   120
    Reverse Back Extensions 122
    Hamstrings Curls   124
    Stiff-legged Deadlifts 126
    Wall Squats   128
    Lunges   130
    Side Lunges   132
    Lateral Leg Raises   134
    Seated Calf Raises   136
Core Concerns: Abs Movements   139
    Abs Crunches (back on the ball) 140
    Abs Crunches (feet on the ball) 142
    Roll-up Crunches   144
    Reverse Crunches   146
    Side Crunches   148
    Cross-body Twists   150
    Side Twists   152
    Hip Raises   154
Be Flexible: Stretches   157
    Back Bend Stretch   158
    Spine Stretch   160
    Side Stretch   162
    Hip Stretch   164
    Roll-out Stretch   166

MOVING FORWARD   **168**
MUSCLE GLOSSARY   **169**
INDEX   **170**
ABOUT THE AUTHOR   **172**

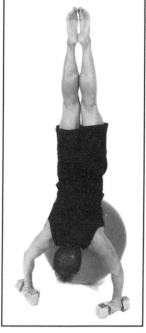

introduction

No matter what your current physical fitness status, you can improve it. It doesn't matter if you're a world-class athlete, a casual exerciser, someone who hasn't exercised for years, someone who's never trained before or someone who is recovering from a serious illness or accident. With the consent of your doctor, when you make the commitment to follow one of the programs in this book, you can get into much better shape than you're currently in.

Regardless of whether you want to look better or improve your health, one of the most beneficial aspects of starting an exercise regimen is that you'll also start to feel better. When you feel better, you'll want to exercise more (or more intensely), and you'll get even better results. You'll start to look firmer; your health markers such as cholesterol, heart rate and body fat levels will start to improve. But most importantly, you'll find that you have more energy. It's ironic that expending more energy is what it takes to have more energy, but that's the nature of the human body. The more demand you place on it, the better able it is to accommodate that demand.

Ulysses Press has asked me to develop this multifaceted exercise program because of a growing awareness and need for a wholesale balance ball and weight-training program. Balance balls have become popular with all levels of exercisers, from first-timers to pro athletes. At first, high-end athletes and body-builders resisted climbing on these brightly colored balls to do what they had been doing on weight benches in weight rooms and gyms. But once a few brave souls risked some name calling, others saw the results these people were getting. Today, balance balls and weights have been integrated into training programs for all sorts of professional sports, and this style of exercise is rapidly spreading into gyms and homes across the country.

Balance ball and weight workouts have been successful because they are both fun and often help people better achieve their goals than traditional weight training alone. Certainly, traditional weight training is a great way to get in shape and build muscle, but integrating balance balls into your weight training helps you improve your ability to train your target muscles while reducing the risk of injury. Though weight training on a balance ball is hard work, it's also a lot of fun. When you sit or lie on the ball, you can feel it move under you—and, after a couple seconds, you can feel your body learning to control the ball, even your first time on the ball. That fast learning curve equates to rapid results, which is exactly what you'll see if you decided to dutifully follow one of the programs in the *Weights on the Ball Workbook*.

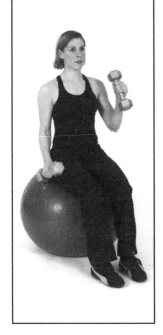

the benefits of "weight"-ing

Patience is a virtue, and so is "weight"-ing. When you train your body with weights, you are doing far more than adding muscle mass for the sake of vanity. Muscle is one indicator of health, and you can never have too much of it. But, first, let me assure you that you will never become more muscular than you want to be. Increased muscle mass doesn't happen by accident—it happens through hard work and diligent pursuit.

It's understandable that many people, particularly women, don't want their bodies to become large and excessively muscular, giving them the bulky appearance that many body-builders have. The programs in this book are designed to allow you to achieve the results you want for your body type, whether you're trying to tone up, reduce body fat or add a little more muscle mass. By choosing the appropriate program and following that workout regimen, you will be able to get the look you're seeking.

Including weight training on the balance ball in your weekly fitness regimen will have numer-ous other positive effects. Your muscle mass will increase regardless of the program you're on, but you won't get that big blocky look—in fact, more mus-cle mass may help you appear smaller than you originally did.

Here's how that works: Muscle mass is denser than fat, and it's possible, particularly if you are on a toning or muscle-building program, that your body will get smaller and tighter. Your body weight may stay the same or even increase a couple pounds, but don't let a small amount of weight gain disturb you—body weight is not a par-ticularly good measure of your fitness level or even your appear-ance. How your clothes fit, how you look in the mirror, and how you appear to others (trust me, they'll notice and they'll compliment you) are far better indicators of the progress you're making on your new *Weights on the Ball* workout.

Adding a few pounds of mus-cle weight may help you weigh less overall. Muscles are very metabolically active, and when you have more muscle mass, your body needs more fuel each day simply to maintain itself. In other words, you burn more calories, even while resting. Couple that with the calories you burn while you perform any of these *Weights on the Ball* programs and you'll find that you have less body fat, increased appetite, and the ability to eat more each day without increasing your body size. And though you may have added a couple pounds of muscle mass, you can easily lose more than that in body fat for a net weight loss. At the same time, your body will become denser and tighter, giving you a more aesthetic and fit appearance.

As you can see, weight training is a win-win situation, as is exercise in general. Couple this with the additional benefits that weight training on a balance ball provide and you, too, can rebuild your body to get the results—and the body—you've always wanted.

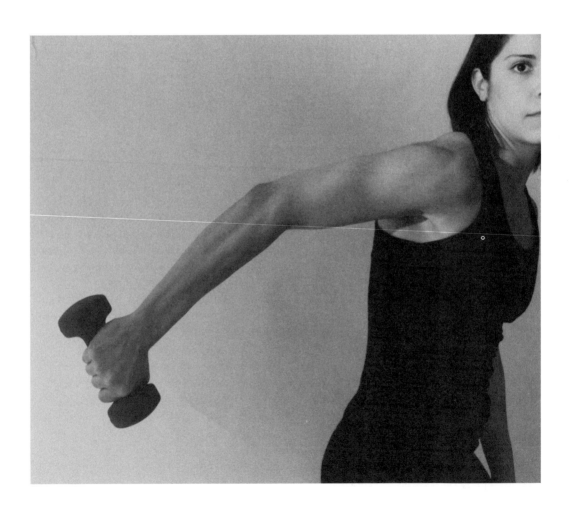

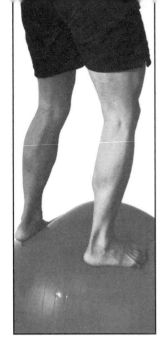

add a little balance to your life

The primary advantage in using a balance ball in your weight training is that it instantly improves your positioning while weight training, and improved positioning will help you better target the muscles you are trying to train in the various exercises.

If you've ever sat on a balance ball, you've probably noticed a couple of things. First, it feels a little wobbly when you first sit down, but after a few seconds you may notice that you begin to stabilize fairly naturally, and it's actually quite comfortable. Second, your posture improves. These two things happen in tandem. As you begin to feel a little unstable, you activate the stabilizer muscles in your body (particularly those in your lower trunk, referred to in this book as your "core").

One of the most effective ways to stabilize your body on the ball is to assume a more proper position. Instead of rounding your lower back, you pull your midsection in a bit and begin to arch your lower back. Now you're sitting more upright with your core held tighter, giving you a longer, leaner look almost instantly.

In time, this positioning and improved posture become more natural, even as you are shedding body fat and adding muscle mass. All these advantages work together to increase your fitness.

These improvements in posture happen regardless of your position on the ball. In fact, in Part Three of the book, where the exercises are detailed, I have grouped the exercises by the position you assume on the ball—for example, seated on the ball, chest on the ball, back on the wall. No matter which position you are in or which muscle you are targeting, you will find that holding your core stable enables you to perform the weight element of the exercise more effectively. The net result is that you not only train your target body part, you also work your midsection by stabilizing during every movement. Regardless of which program you are on, having a tighter midsection will enhance your goal, your level of fitness and your overall appearance.

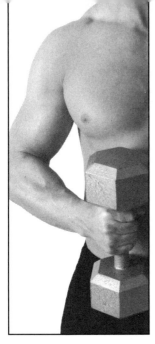

muscle matters

The body is made up of muscle groups that are composed of major, minor and stabilizer muscles. For the purposes of this book, I'll be referring primarily to major muscle groups and stabilizers. The major muscle groups of the body include shoulders, back, chest, triceps, biceps and legs. Abdominals are also a muscle group, but I'll often refer to them as "core" muscles—all those of the lower trunk, both front and back, not just the six-pack, or rectus abdominis muscle. For more extensive definitions of muscles and terminology, please turn to the Muscle Glossary at the end of the book.

Your major muscle groups also consist of minor muscles, stabilizers and assisting muscles, which help when you target certain muscle groups. Your goal is to get your target muscle group to do as much work as possible. By using your stabilizers and holding your core tight, you can rely more on the target muscle and less on assisting muscles.

For example, when you perform a chest press (pages 68–69) with your back on the ball, you want to hold your core tight and press the weight up using your

pecs (with a little assistance from your triceps). If you perform the rep incorrectly by allowing your midsection to be loose and mobile, you will feel the movement of the weight in your entire upper body since you are forced to use more of your shoulder muscles to compensate for your weak positioning. This is not biomechanically sound and can potentially lead to injury, particularly if this sloppy type of movement becomes a habit. Using a weight you can comfort-

ably control while holding your core tight will allow you to avoid injury *and* more effectively develop your chest muscles. Since you will also be doing the same when you train your shoulders—holding your core tight as you target your delts—there is no advantage in allowing assisting muscle groups to do more work than needed during chest movements.

The same holds true for all body parts. Strive to work your major target muscles and try to reduce the work of assisting muscles. By stabilizing with your core and other stabilizer muscles, you will drive the effort into the muscle group you are trying to target. This is much easier to do on a ball than it is to do on a weight bench because the bench does much of the stabilizing for you. By performing the same routine on a balance ball, you can actually work your target muscles more readily, making it easier to achieve your goals. This is one of the big benefits that these weights-on-the-ball programs have over basic weight-training programs.

Regardless of how you weight-train your muscles or what your intended goal is, you must allow your muscles a certain amount of recovery. Muscles don't grow because they are weight-trained; they grow because they recover from weight training. Providing a muscle with the stimulation of weights sends that muscle the message that it must adapt to the greater demand you're placing on it. After you finish your workout, your body will spend the next several days repairing the stress damage that you've inflicted on it (this "damage" isn't harmful—often it's barely noticeable; at other times, you may recognize it, essentially, as the soreness that comes after training).

Allowing each body part a couple days to a week of recovery is built into the workout schedule charts for each program. Notice that muscle-building programs give individual body parts more time to recover—this is because muscle grows best with intense stimulation and relatively long periods of recovery. For toning and slimming programs, you often work the same body part more than once a week. This is fine since you do not stimulate individual muscle groups to exhaustion in individual sessions; thus, they do not need as much recovery time before they are ready to work again.

Muscle is an amazing commodity—certainly worth its weight in gold. As you begin to accumulate more of it from your *Weights on the Ball* workout, you'll fully appreciate how valuable it is.

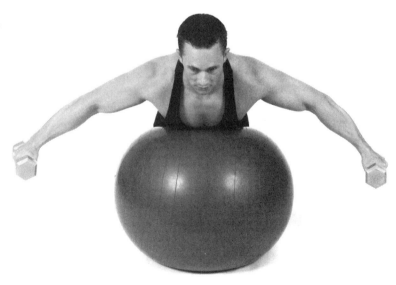

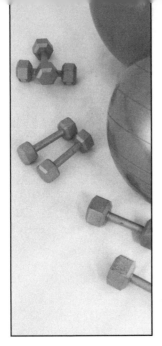

equipped for success

For these weights-on-the-ball workouts, all you need to get started is a balance ball, a pair of dumbbells and the time to train. I've also included some extras that will help you more fully train your whole body. Here's a breakdown of the equipment you'll need.

The Ball

These brightly colored orbs are known by a variety of different names, including exercise balls, stability balls, Swiss balls and balance balls. I prefer to call them balance balls because that's how I think of them in my workouts, and the term "balance ball" is nice and alliterative.

These balls first gained popularity with specialty exercise such as rehab and sport-specific training, but they are rapidly moving into the mainstream; it's hard to find a gym without one these days. They are quite durable and safe—I've never seen one burst, although they do occasionally develop slow leaks. While you can patch a leak, if the ball continues to deflate, it's time to replace it. Nevertheless, the average ball should give you months, if not years, of performance.

Balance balls come in a variety of colors and sizes (and prices). You can spend up to about $50 for the largest, most durable balls. If you find a price that's higher than this, I recommend you keep looking. For high-end balls, try such stores as Relax the Back Store, or look online at such websites as www.sitincomfort.com.

Choosing your first ball can be a little tricky. The basic recommendation is to choose a ball that you can comfortably sit on, as so many of the exercises from the various workouts rely on that position. If you're shorter than 5' 3", choose a 55 cm ball; if you fall between 5' 3" and 6', go with a 65 cm ball; and if you're taller, you might opt for a 75 cm ball.

Use the following as a rule of thumb for gauging whether a ball is the right size for basic movements: When you sit on a ball, near the center, your upper legs should be about parallel to the ground. The ball should be inflated so that it still gives a bit under the pressure of your weight. To know if the ball is properly inflated, hold the ball and squeeze it between your palms; it should change shape a bit, getting a little flatter. If the ball resists you too much and you are of reasonable strength, then the ball is inflated too much for the purposes of the workouts in this book. You can let out a little air.

There is no one perfect ball for all exercises. You're better off having a couple of different ones. I'm 5' 8", and I have a 65 and 75 cm ball. I find that the 65 cm is best for seated movements, but when I need a little more size with the ball, the 75 cm provides that; plus, advanced moves (such as the kneeling version of seated moves, see page 55) are a little easier—albeit scarier—on the big ball.

The Weights

As with the ball, you're probably going to want more than one pair of dumbbells, but it's perfectly fine to start with just one. My recommendation is to opt for a slightly lighter rather than heavier first set. If you choose a heavier weight, you may not be able to perform certain exercises (for instance, if you have a weaker upper body, you may not be able to press as much weight as you can use for leg movements such as wall squats). But if you choose a lighter set of weights, you'll be able to perform every exercise.

As you add to your weight arsenal, you can choose to buy a few different sets of dumbbells. If you don't consider yourself to be very strong, you might start with a pair of dumbbells in the two- to five-pound range. If you're reasonably strong, five to ten pounds may still allow you to complete all (or most) of the exercises in the program you choose to follow. Make your best estimate, choosing lighter rather than heavier.

Then, as you make progress, you can start buying pairs of dumbbells in heavier increments. Often, weight trainers (and women in particular) grow very comfortable using the same

weight every time they train. It's invigorating to be able to perform your workout rapidly and easily. The only problem is that you won't continue to make gains the way you did initially. Adding a little weight is one of the best ways to keep improving. You'll notice that our dark-haired model, Andrea, puts up some pretty big weights, but notice how toned and thin her arms are. She frequently trains with heavier weights, and it hasn't made her thick or blocky. In fact, she continues to make improvements. Today, she looks taller and thinner than when I first started training with her a couple of years ago. So let me reiterate: I like to see female weight trainers push a decent amount of weight. It really helps you accomplish your goals.

The Accessories

While you clearly can't perform a weights and ball workout without weights and a ball, the following pieces of equipment are optional. Choosing to use them will make your workouts more versatile and effective, but you can certainly achieve your goals with substitutes as well.

Weight Bench

A weight bench can be useful in many exercises. For moves where your hands or feet are on the ball, you can often place the other on a bench. In addition, you can often use a weight bench for stability, placing the

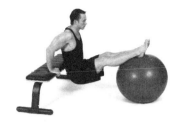

A weight bench can be useful in many exercises.

ball against the bench for challenging exercises.

At home, if you do not have a weight bench available, often you can find a substitute, such as a couch, a chair or other stable piece of furniture. Improvising can help make your workout much more versatile if you don't have the accessories on this list.

Ankle Weights

While these are not necessary for the program, ankle weights can be beneficial because you simply strap them on to your ankles or wrists. This makes certain movements easier because you don't have to hold the dumbbells, particularly for some of the tricky movements such as hamstrings curls (see page 124). Consider purchasing a pair or two (of differing weight) for these moves.

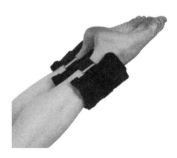

Ankle weights.

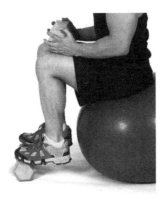

Using a weight in place of a block.

Block for Raises

For certain movements, it's best to elevate your body off the ground a bit. A yoga block or any other stable block is ideal for this (you may also be able to use the bottom step of a stairway). Our solution was to use one of the weights as a block, but notice that the weight we used has flat surfaces on the head. Do not use a round weight for this move as it could potentially lead to injury.

Mats

You may feel more secure if you place a mat under your ball for certain movements. A mat will often make the ball a little more stable since it often creates a little more friction than the surface of your floor. We used yoga mats several times during the balance ball photo shoot. Often, a yoga mat can provide you with a little more traction to help create more stability. Finally, mats provide a little padding in the event of a balance mishap. Balance mishaps, like wardrobe malfunctions, can happen when you least expect them. Having a mat underneath you can help alleviate the pain, if not the humiliation.

A Wall

You may not typically think of a wall as a piece of exercise equipment, but as you read through the exercise descriptions and variations, you may notice how we've worked it into the various programs. Often, placing the ball or a part of your body against a wall is helpful or even crucial to performing an exercise. For example, you simply couldn't perform wall squats without one! And this is such a great exercise for building and toning leg muscles that it warrants including an open space of wall as a piece of equipment. *Note:* If all the wall space in your home is filled with furniture, you can substitute a closed door as your wall.

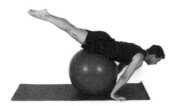

A yoga mat provides traction to help create more stability.

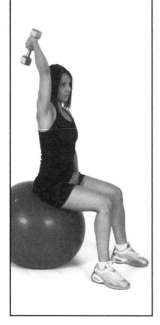

form and effort

When working out, the better form you use to execute each rep and the more effort you put into each rep, the better your results will be. In my years of experience, there are two major mistakes I see being committed virtually every time I go to the gym. One mistake is more typical of men, the other is more typical of women (see if you can tell which is which). Please take the information in this section to heart and eliminate both of these mistakes from your own training. You'll get better results and be far less likely to injure yourself.

Mistakes

1) **Performing reps on remote control.** Every rep you perform should be purposeful and thoughtful, with your full concentration placed on it. When you put yourself on autopilot and merely perform a set number of reps, usually a high number with a light weight, you aren't working your muscles as hard as you should. Often, your muscles are barely working at all as you are able to use your joints for leverage. In addition, this leads to sloppy movement, where you don't take the weights through their most effective range of motion to really work the muscle that you want to target. It can also lead to injury since you are working your joints more than your muscles, and not necessarily through the range of motion that they were designed to move through. This is a common mistake made by many women (though quite a few men do the same).

2) **Using too much weight and cheating.** Okay, this is usually a male mistake. Men often have the idea that others are looking at how much weight they are using. To try to avoid embarrassment, many guys choose a weight that is too heavy for them, and they struggle, twist, grunt and contort trying to perform a rep. Guess what draws more attention than using a light weight? A noisy spastic begging someone to pull the weight off his chest. Even if you can get the weight up on your own, if you aren't able to do it by targeting the muscle you are intending to work, then you are using too much weight.

Solutions—Perfect Your Reps

To get the most from your program, you want to choose a

weight that reasonably allows you to perform all the reps of a given set at the indicated effort level without breaking form.

Throughout the exercise descriptions, I emphasize the stretch and the contraction on each rep. This advice can be easy to ignore, but I implore you to follow it if you want to get the most from your program. Do me a favor and follow along with my description of performing a rep right now, and see if you can't feel the difference:

First, extend your arm all the way until it's straight and make a fist. From that position, begin to raise your lower arm, keeping your upper arm stationary. Squeeze your biceps (along the front of your upper arm). Take three to five seconds to bring your lower arm up until your fist is near your shoulder. Contract your biceps good and hard at the top and hold that for about two seconds. Now, continuing to hold your upper arm stationary and continuing to tense your biceps, begin to lower the lower part of your arm (with your hand still in a fist), feeling a stretch along the top of your biceps. Take about three seconds to lower your arm until your arm is fully extended. Perform three more reps like that before you read on.

After only four of these reps (up to 10 seconds for each), your biceps should feel much warmer and fatigued than it did before you did this modest exercise. This is because you just executed these reps with perfect form and full effort. Think how much more taxed your target muscle will feel when you use weight, and think how much better your results will be.

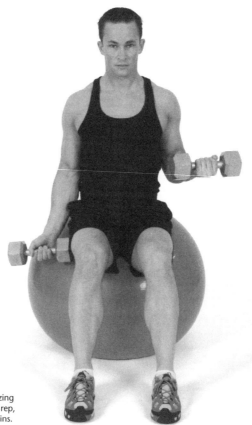

When you use strict form, emphasizing the stretch and contraction of each rep, you'll significantly improve your gains.

warming up and stretching

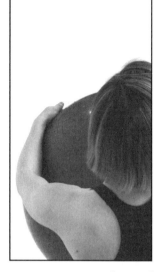

People often confuse "warm-ups" and "stretching," believing them to be the same thing. In actuality, they are two separate activities, but both are often performed at the beginning of a workout. Regardless of the type of workout you perform, it's a great idea to warm up first in order to circulate your blood and to raise your body temperature. One way to do this is to walk with purpose or to use a piece of cardio equipment such as a treadmill, stair stepper or stationary bike for six to ten minutes before you begin your workout. Keep your pace moderate, and just focus on bringing up your core temperature.

Once you have raised your core temperature, this is an ideal time to stretch before exercising. Your muscles are a little warmer and much more pliable than they were before your warm up. At this point, you're much less likely to injure yourself from stretching tight muscles.

It's a good idea to take your body through the range of motion that you will use for every exercise in your workout that day. For each movement, perform a few reps without any weight, slightly exaggerating the motion that you'll use. You can also use the ball to perform stretches (see pages 157–67), or improvise and perform personal favorite stretches on the ball or on the floor.

Keep in mind that stretching, too, is exercise: if you want to stretch intensely, the best time to do this is after your weight workout or on a day when you're not performing your *Weights on the Ball* workout, not directly before your workout. That's for intense stretching.

A warm-up stretch, however, is different and should be performed after your warm-up and before your workout. A "warm-up stretch" need not last longer than about five minutes; you don't want to stretch your muscles to their limits as this may undercut their ability to stretch and contract when you perform your weight workout.

So at the start of your workout, keep it simple. Perform a short warm up, then include a short warm-up stretch. Ideally, you should do both, but I realize that time is short and often you'll want to get right to your *Weights on the Ball* workout. In this case, I recommend doing a warm-up weight set, where you use considerably less weight for the first set of each exercise than you do for the regular sets that follow. This warm-up set will help increase the temperature of your target muscle, help you get accustomed to the feeling of the movement, and ultimately help you better train it with less risk of injury.

In fact, on days when time permits, you can perform more than one warm-up set, "pyramiding" up in weight until you reach the weight for your first working set. For instance, let's say that your working weight is 15 pounds. You might first perform a warm-up set with 5 pounds, then a second with 1 0 pounds. Now you are primed to perform your working sets at 15 pounds. Perform the number of sets listed on the chart in your program, and don't count those warm-ups toward your working sets!

Additionally, I like to perform a warm-up set with a lighter weight for each subsequent exercise, too. Include these if your schedule allows for the time these will take.

Warming up and stretching are essential parts of exercising. Often, people don't include them and then suffer injuries or unnecessary soreness. Many times, this mindset comes from our memories of being 18, when our bodies were ready to go at a second's notice. As you pass that milestone (and who hasn't?), take into account the changes that your body has undergone. Treat your body right by warming up and stretching as much as you feel your body needs.

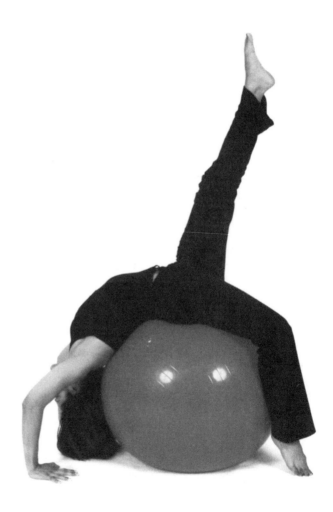

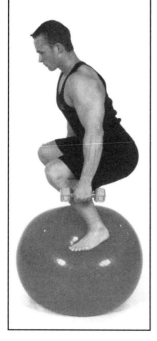

cardio concerns

I've written this book because I believe that working out with weights on the ball is one of the most fun and effective ways to achieve your fitness goals. However, cardiovascular exercise—such as walking, jogging, jumping rope or even working on a piece of equipment such as a treadmill, stair stepper or stationary bike—is beneficial: it improves your heart health, general level of fitness and your ability to get results from other forms of exercise.

Since you've just recently purchased a book about weight training on a stability ball, you probably aren't seeking a cardiovascular program that is based on increasing your heart rate and raising your body temperature. Nevertheless—there's always a nevertheless, isn't there?—including some cardio exercise in your overall fitness program will only enhance the results you get from weight training on a balance ball.

You may be surprised to learn that you can use the ball to perform cardiovascular exercise. In several of the programs, I rec-

ommend "circuit training," where you perform a large number of reps (usually 20 to 30) of one exercise before moving directly into the next exercise. Targeting larger muscles such as the legs with high reps really increases the cardiovascular work you must do, and performing cardiovascular exercise with light weights for these high reps on your balance ball allows you to have your cake and eat it, too.

Still, I'd be remiss if I didn't recommend that you include at least two sessions of cardiovascular work a week, even if it's

just walking with purpose for 20 minutes or so to get your body warm and your heart rate up a bit. The best times to do cardio are after you perform your weights or first thing in the morning, but other times of the day are fine, too.

In the sample schedules provided with the various programs in Part Two, I've noted days on which to perform cardio. Please try to fit them into your schedule as best as you can. While cardiovascular training is not a requirement of these programs, you'll find that it will help you attain your goals more rapidly.

part two:

programmed for success

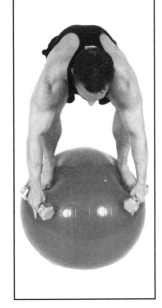

let's get personal: an overview

No matter your experience, skill level or goals, you'll get the results you're seeking if you follow the program that's right for you. The programs in this book target many different readers and their individual needs. *Firm Foundation* teaches you how to get toned; *Slim and Trim* addresses the exercise needs for those whose primary goal is burning body fat; *Muscle Bound* explains the strategies for adding muscle mass.

Read through the opening descriptions of each of these programs to decide which is right for you, then use the guidance provided to help you get started. Start slowly and build up to the level of exercise and fitness you want to attain. For instance, you may start with the Firm Foundation Level 1 workout. But after a month or two of training, you may feel you can do more and want to move on to Level 2 or Level 3. That's part of the thought process beyond these programs—I'd like to see you do a little more exercise each week as your fitness level improves.

Then, after you've been on your program for a while—usually two or four months of regular exercise, progressing through the levels of your program—you can become more creative and start modifying your program (see "Moving Forward" at the end of the book).

Above all, pick a program—and exercises—that seems like it will be fun for you. When you enjoy what you're doing, you're much more likely to keep doing it. This type of consistency is what really leads to the results you're seeking.

Program Basics

With each program, I've included a workout schedule that gives you one way to incorporate your training program into your daily life. But I also realize that one size does not fit all. Some people like to work out in the mornings. Others don't like to exercise at that time of day, but can only do it then. Still others prefer to work out in the evenings after work, or even later, after the kids are in bed.

Whatever your preferences or needs, you can build any of these programs into your life in ways that differ from the set program schedule included in each workout. Just keep the following tips in mind if you need to customize one of the programs to you personal needs:

• **In general, try not to group rest days together in big blocks.** One of the benefits of regular exercise is that you are constantly stimulating the metabolic rate of your body. As such, if you're going to work out three days a week, it's better to work out on Monday, Wednesday and Friday (or Tuesday, Thursday and Saturday) than it is to work out three days in a row and then take four days in a row off as you wait for your next week's exercise cycle to come around.

You also may not work out as hard by that third day in a row, as your body feels the effects of accumulated fatigue. Giving yourself a rest day between workout days allows your body to repair and regroup so that it's ready for the next workout. My workout schedules take this into account, but they may not work for your life schedule. Go ahead and change up the days and times so that they better fit your life.

• **Recognize your individual goal when building your schedule.** The programs I've designed specifically target the goal of that section. For instance, the Slim and Trim workouts emphasize larger muscle groups (such as legs) over smaller muscle group (such as biceps or triceps) because working these large groups burns more calories and better stimulates the fat-burning process. However, the Muscle Bound program works one muscle group hard during one workout, then allows it several days to recover. Since muscle grows during periods of rest after stimulation, this is a key component to success in the Muscle Bound program. It's important for you to recognize the strategies for achieving your particular goal. That way, if you need to make modifications to your program, you can do so while still incorporating these strategies into any changes you might make.

• **If you miss a workout, don't beat yourself up about it.** Often, people are too hard on themselves when they miss a workout. They decide that they have failed, and this can lead to giving up the program altogether. A missed workout or two is no big deal. Just get back on your program as soon as you can, and don't worry about what you missed. Some is always better than none. If time doesn't permit you to do a full workout, then just do ten minutes. Or five minutes. Again, some is always better than none.

• **Soreness is normal; excessive soreness is not.** When you work out, especially after a long layoff, it's normal to expect to feel a little sore, especially the next day and the day after you work out. I'd rather have you start slowly and be a little less sore after your first workouts. At first, err on the side of a little less rather than a little more, taking your current fitness status into account. When you feel soreness from exercise, you really should only notice it when you move. If you feel any aches or pains while you are stationary, this is an indications of excessive soreness or potential injury. Should this happen to you, consult a physician to see if you need additional medical attention.

Choosing your weight level

The amount of weight you'll use differs depending on the program you're on, as you'll see. Please refer to the weight level chart in order to determine your own personal weight levels.

WEIGHT LEVEL CHART	
1 WARM-UP	A weight that you can perform reps with indefinitely, working well beyond the rep ranges for your program.
2 LIGHT	A weight where you can easily perform all the reps within your rep range.
3 MODERATE	A weight where you feel moderate fatigue as you reach the end of your rep range.
4 HEAVY	A weight where you feel fatigue such that you need to rest at least a minute before performing your next set.
5 FAILURE	A weight where you are not able to perform another rep in that set (but that does allow you to still reach the rep range).

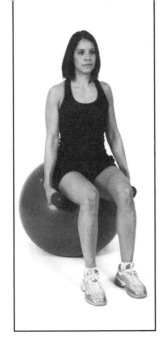

firm foundation

Whether you're a beginning exerciser, or someone who has had a long lay off from exercise (due to a career, children or other demands of life), or even if you're a senior who has had little experience with exercise, this is an excellent beginning point. This program addresses the needs of those who are interested in toning up their bodies. Of course, most people (even some professional athletes!) might say they would like to have a better toned body.

For the purposes of this book, and to help you evaluate whether this program is the right one for you in this book, I am defining "toning" as tightening up your body without making a radical shift in your body composition (or body weight, although I'm a little loathe to use this as a parameter). This means that you're relatively happy with your body size, and you're most interested in looking and feeling a little better, and you recognize that exercise with weights will help you achieve this goal.

Of course, you must talk to your doctor to make certain that

an exercise regimen such as this is right for you—all forms of exercise place demands on the body, and you must have the requisite health for this. If your body is not yet ready for a Level 1 toning workout with weights on the ball, you may need to work with a medical professional, physical therapist or trainer to help you get to this stage.

Once you have clearance from your doctor, start slowly with Level 1. Think of this program—and all its sets, reps and exercises—as the first goal that you are working toward. You don't have to perform every

exercise for every set and rep the first time. Work within your limits at the beginning, and progress slowly. The goal is to become a regular exerciser, to get in shape and stay in shape. And that doesn't happen by performing a few arduous sessions from the start. That mindset can make you excessively sore, which will certainly undercut your enjoyment (and, in the long run, the benefits of the program). So enjoy yourself and don't overdo it!

Level 2 and Level 3 in this toning program are for those who are used to a moderate amount of exercise, and who

FIRM FOUNDATION: BODY TONING		
	SCHEDULE	PROGRAM DESCRIPTION
LEVEL 1	2 times a week; 20–30 min./session	For new or returning exercisers who have limited time but want to firm up their bodies.
LEVEL 2	3 times a week; 20–30 min./session	For those who have a little more time for exercise and want to see even greater toning results.
LEVEL 3	3 times a week; 45 min./session	For fit individuals who want to achieve a fit and toned appearance, and have the time to do so.

have the time to devote at least three days a week to exercise (20–30 minutes for Level 2; 45 minutes for Level 3). If you are already at this level, give Level 2 a try before jumping up to Level 3. After a couple of weeks at Level 2, you may be ready to advance to working with weights for 45 minutes three times a week. I think this is a reasonable exercise goal for healthy adults of all ages. I'd like to encourage everyone to set this as a goal and start working towards it, but do so at your own pace.

Getting the most out of your workout

Regardless of which level you choose in this program, for more cardiovascular training, you can perform a set of one exercise, then move on to the next exercise, performing one set of each exercise. Rest as little as possible between sets. Then, return to the first exercise and perform a second round, continuing until you've performed all reps of all sets. This type of circuit training will help keep your heart rate up and promote fat burning

and heart health while you tone up.

On the other hand, if you're more interested in building a little more muscle, then perform all the sets of one exercise before moving onto the next. Take a short rest period between sets (about 30 seconds) to allow your muscles to recover, then begin the next set of the same exercise. After completing all sets of this exercise, move on to the next exercise.

Weight levels

For all levels in this program, start with a level 1 weight and work up through weight levels 2 and 3 until you are able to perform all sets and reps with level 3 weights. Those who are already conditioned can begin with level 2 or 3 weights, depending on their fitness and strength. See the chart on page 19 for an overview to the levels.

firm foundation: level 1
twice a week for 20–30 minutes

If you only have enough time to work out twice a week and you're limited by how much time you can devote during each session (either by your conditioning or by your busy schedule), it's a good idea to include both upper- and lower-body work during each session.

This program also makes slight adjustments from Workout One to Workout Two so that you are stimulating your upper and lower body in a different way each workout. This strategy allows you to work many of the major muscles of your entire body twice a week, and encourages better overall toning than performing the same workout every time you train.

The objective of each workout is to accomplish as much as you can in this short allotment of time. As your conditioning improves, try to reduce the amount of time that you rest between sets. This will increase the cardiovascular demands you place on your body, enhancing endurance and overall fitness as well as helping you to tone your muscles.

WEEKLY SCHEDULE	
MONDAY	Workout 1
TUESDAY	20 min. cardio
WEDNESDAY	rest
THURSDAY	Workout 2
FRIDAY	20 min. cardio
SATURDAY	rest
SUNDAY	rest

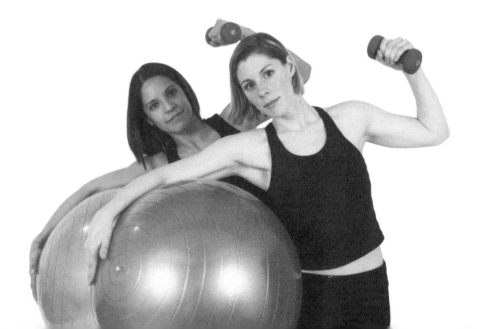

FIRM FOUNDATION: LEVEL 1

workout 1

PAGE	EXERCISE	TARGET	SETS	REPS
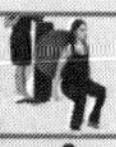 128	wall squats	legs	3	15–20
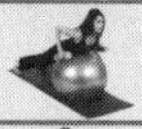 96	dumbbell rows (chest on ball)	back	2	15
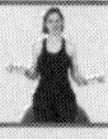 50	alternate biceps curls	biceps	2	15
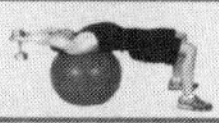 76	pullovers	back	2	12
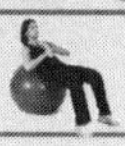 140	abs crunches (back on ball)	abs	2	15

workout 2

PAGE	EXERCISE	TARGET	SETS	REPS
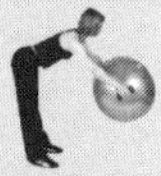 126	stiff-legged deadlifts	hamstrings, glutes, lower back	3	15–20
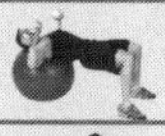 68	flat chest presses	chest	2	15
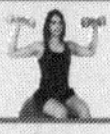 60	shoulder presses	shoulders	2	15
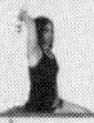 54	triceps extensions (seated)	triceps	2	15
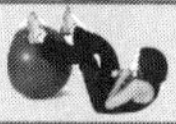 142	abs crunches (feet on ball)	abs	2	15

firm foundation: level 2
three times a week for 20–30 minutes

Even though you have time to do three workouts a week, I have provided only two separate workouts. The way you should proceed is to perform Workout One first, then Workout Two second. You're third workout of the week will be to repeat Workout One. The next week, start with Workout Two, so that you simply alternate these two workouts, training a total of three times a week. This strategy will allow you to work all the parts of your body at least three times every two weeks. (See the sample schedules.)

If the amount of time that you can devote to exercising increases, you can add reps to the exercises included in these workouts (but don't do more than 20). Once you are performing three sets of each of these exercises, you can begin to add new exercises to the mix. Choose those you would like to try, or those that target body areas you are most interested in improving. (See "Moving Forward" at the end of the book for more suggestions.)

WEEK ONE	
MONDAY	Workout 1
TUESDAY	20 min. cardio
WEDNESDAY	Workout 2
THURSDAY	rest
FRIDAY	Workout 1
SATURDAY	20 min. cardio
SUNDAY	rest

WEEK TWO	
MONDAY	Workout 2
TUESDAY	20 min. cardio
WEDNESDAY	Workout 1
THURSDAY	rest
FRIDAY	Workout 2
SATURDAY	20 min. cardio
SUNDAY	rest

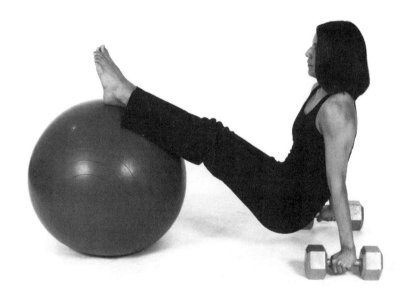

FIRM FOUNDATION: LEVEL 2

workout 1

	PAGE	EXERCISE	TARGET	SETS	REPS
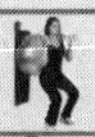	128	wall squat curls	legs, biceps	3	15–20
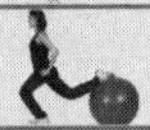	130	lunges	legs	2	12
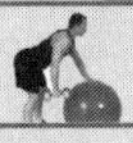	104	dumbbell rows (hand on ball)	back	2	15
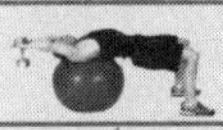	76	pullovers	chest, back	2	12
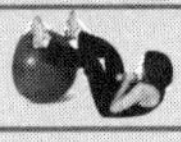	142	abs crunches (feet on ball)	abs	2	15

workout 2

	PAGE	EXERCISE	TARGET	SETS	REPS
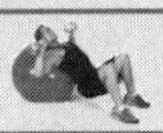	70	incline chest presses	chest	3	15
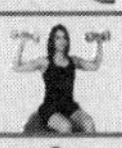	60	shoulder presses	shoulders	2	15
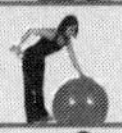	102	triceps kickbacks (hand on ball)	triceps	2	15
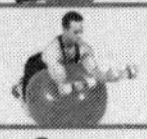	90	preacher curls	biceps	2	15
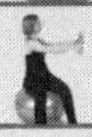	152	side twists	abs, obliques	2	15

firm foundation: level 3
three times a week for 45 minutes

This is a thorough, full-body program designed to promote ultimate toning. If that's your goal and you have the time to devote to it, I recommend that you think of this program as your goal, even if your starting fitness level doesn't allow you to do this workout yet.

Perform Workout One first, then Workout Two second. Your third workout of the week is to repeat Workout One and then start the second week with Workout Two. (See the sample schedules on the next page.) This will allow you

WEEK ONE	
MONDAY	Workout 1
TUESDAY	20 min. cardio
WEDNESDAY	Workout 2
THURSDAY	rest
FRIDAY	Workout 1
SATURDAY	20 min. cardio
SUNDAY	rest

WEEK TWO	
MONDAY	Workout 2
TUESDAY	20 min. cardio
WEDNESDAY	Workout 1
THURSDAY	rest
FRIDAY	Workout 2
SATURDAY	20 min. cardio
SUNDAY	rest

to train all body parts three times in two weeks.

Above all, keep it moving when you perform this toning workout. Try not to rest for very long between sets unless you are

winded or fatigued. When you exercise in a more continuous fashion, this enhances the cardiovascular element of your training, encouraging better overall fitness and toning.

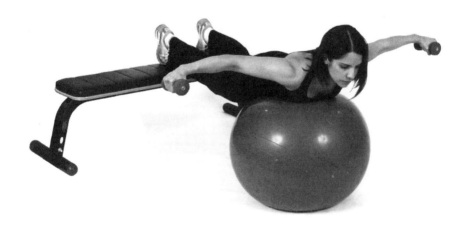

firm foundation 3

workout 1

	PAGE	EXERCISE	TARGET	SETS	REPS
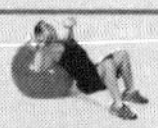	70	incline chest presses	chest	3	15
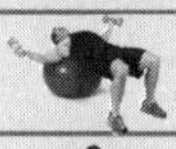	72	flat chest flyes	chest	3	15
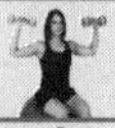	60	shoulder presses	shoulders	3	15
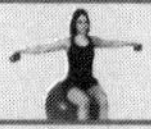	58	lateral raises	shoulders	3	15
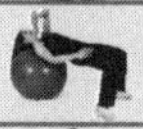	78	triceps extensions (back on ball)	triceps	3	15
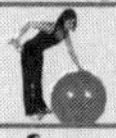	102	triceps kickbacks (hand on ball)	triceps	3	15
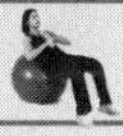	140	abs crunches (back on ball)	abs	3	15

workout 2

	PAGE	EXERCISE	TARGET	SETS	REPS
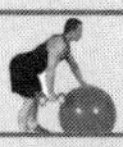	104	dumbbell rows (hand on ball)	back	3	15
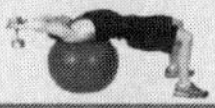	76	pullovers	back	3	12
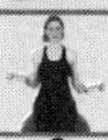	50	alternate biceps curls	biceps	3	15
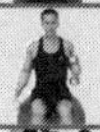	52	hammer curls	biceps	3	15
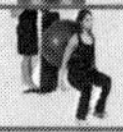	128	wall squats	legs	3	15
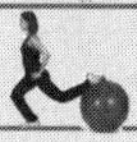	130	lunges	legs	3	15

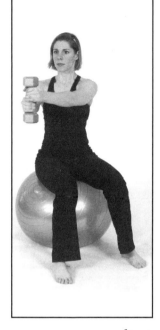

slim and trim

If your goal is to reduce body fat, then this is the program for you. The more time you can devote to exercise (within reason), the faster you'll see results. In addition to exercise, you should work to make adjustments in your nutrition program. I like the phrase "nutrition program" because it's a much more accurate and far more palatable phrase than "diet."

When you want to burn body fat, the equation is simple on the surface—you need to take in fewer calories than you burn each day. Those calories that you burn but do not replace with food must still be supplied by your body. They will be pulled from storage and used as energy. This program is designed to help you pull stored energy from body fat. One of the risks of crash diets or rigorous exercise programs is that they often break down muscle mass to use as energy over stored body fat. When you lose muscle, you end up lowering your metabolic rate, which ultimately makes it even easier for your body to add more fat, even if you don't increase the amount of food you consume.

Getting the most out of your workout
The techniques described in this program will help you keep your muscle mass while encouraging the loss of body fat. Here are a few strategies that all the programs in this chapter are based upon.

First, work your biggest muscles groups frequently. Every time you work out, you should work your lower body. Working this largest muscle group in the body burns more calories while at the same time stimulates these muscles to grow. Your goal is not to make your legs large; it's to increase muscle mass enough to raise your metabolic rate so that you are pulling fat from storage for energy.

Second, work your upper body, too. By stimulating your whole body every time you work out, you're encouraging overall muscle growth and upping the amount of calories you're burning. Often, weight trainers overemphasize either upper- or lower-body training at the expense of the other. It's much better to work both in each workout when trying to reduce body fat.

Third, incorporate cardiovascular training with your weight training. It doesn't matter what type of cardiovascular exercise

SLIM AND TRIM: DECREASING BODY FAT		
	SCHEDULE	**PROGRAM DESCRIPTION**
LEVEL 1	2 times a week; 20–30 min./session	For new or returning exercisers who have limited time but want to reduce their body fat levels.
LEVEL 2	3 times a week; 20–30 min./session	For those who have a little more time for exercise and want to devote more time and effort to reducing body fat.
LEVEL 3	3 times a week; 45 min./session	For individuals with the fitness level and time to devote to a full, fat-reducing exercise regimen.

you do as long as you enjoy it enough that you'll do it regularly. See "Cardio Concerns" (page 15) for some ideas. Walking is one of the best forms of exercise, and it's easy to incorporate into your life. Even if you don't have 20 or 30 minutes to set aside for it every day, try to walk as much as possible as you perform your daily routine. Walking when you first get up in the morning for a half hour, or 20 minutes, or even 10, can really help jumpstart your day and get your body going. (You can do this on an empty stomach, and your body will tap into fat stores when it starts searching for energy to replenish itself.)

Often, it takes your body a few weeks to reverse the storing process and start burning body fat. Give it the opportunity to work and don't get discouraged. Also, don't focus too much on your body weight. Since you are also trying to add a little muscle mass, your net weight loss is not the best measure of your success. Focus more on the

way you appear and how your clothes fit. If you notice the ratio of your upper body to midsection improving, then that means you are on the road to success.

This chapter presents three levels for you to choose from. The primary factors in helping you decide where to start are: 1) Your current fitness level, and 2) The amount of time you have to devote to your weights-on-the ball training program.

Level 1 is a beginner's program in which you work out twice a week for no more than 30 minutes. It's a great place to start, especially if you have not been exercising recently (or ever). If the demands of this level are beyond your current fitness level, do what you can. You can increase the rest time a bit between sets. Give your body the opportunity to slowly adapt to the increased demands you're asking of it. You'll find this is a better strategy than forcing it to do too much.

To really begin to see fat-burning success, I think it's a

much better strategy to perform your weights-on-the-ball routine three times a week. Level 2 provides three separate weekly workouts to help you raise your metabolic rate and really start burning body fat.

As your fitness level improves, and if your schedule allows for it, Level 3 is the best way to burn body fat at a reasonably fast rate. Training for up to 45 minutes, three times a week, with weights and the balance ball is an ideal strategy for burning body fat. Again, it's reasonable to target this workout as your goal and build up to it slowly. Give your body the opportunity to adapt to your workout regimen and you'll see fast results without the miserable side effects (excessive soreness, potential injury) that often accompany over-estimating your body's abilities.

Weight levels

Beginners should start with level 1 weights, working up to and through level 2 and 3 weights. Ultimately, in the second and third levels of this program, I'd like to see some level 4 weights incorporated, although you don't need to do that for each set. Eventually, you should strive to complete your last set of each exercise with a level 4 weight. See the chart on page 19 for an overview to the levels.

slim and trim: level 1
twice a week for 20–30 minutes

The objective of this fat-burning program is two-fold: 1) To introduce your body to exercise. If you have not exercised before, or are returning after a long hiatus, don't overdo it. Get clearance from a doctor and don't feel you have to perform all of this program if your body is not quite ready. 2) To allow you to reduce your body fat while maintaining a busy lifestyle that doesn't allow much time for exercise.

Each of the two workouts here should be performed once a week. You can perform these exercises in a circuit rotation, doing the first set of the first exercise, followed by the first set of the second exercise, and so on

until you reach the end of the circuit. Then go back through until you have completed all the sets of the workout.

If you prefer, though, you can also perform all the sets for the first exercise before moving on to the second exercise. This strategy stimulates your target muscles a little more, but may take you longer as you need to rest a bit longer between sets.

Note that both workouts start with "wall squat curls," a great time saver. Simply perform wall squats and simultaneously curl dumbbells in each hand up toward your shoulders as you lower your body. If time allows, you can replace this movement

WEEKLY SCHEDULE	
MONDAY	Workout 1
TUESDAY	20 min. cardio
WEDNESDAY	rest
THURSDAY	Workout 2
FRIDAY	20 min. cardio
SATURDAY	rest
SUNDAY	rest

with regular wall squats and seated biceps curls.

If this workout proves too taxing in the beginning, you don't have to complete it all. Reduce the number of sets, reps or exercises and build up until you can comfortably perform the entire workout.

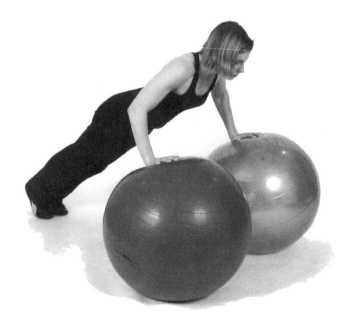

SLIM AND TRIM: LEVEL 1

workout 1

	PAGE	EXERCISE	TARGET	SETS	REPS
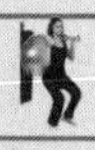	128	wall squat curls	legs, biceps	3	20
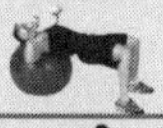	68	flat chest presses	chest	2	20
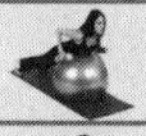	96	dumbbell rows (chest on ball)	back	2	20
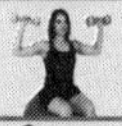	60	shoulder presses	shoulders	2	20
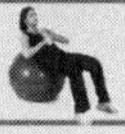	140	abs crunches (back on ball)	abs	2	15

workout 2

	PAGE	EXERCISE	TARGET	SETS	REPS
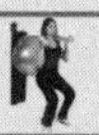	128	wall squat curls	legs, biceps	3	20
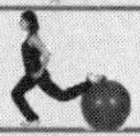	130	lunges	legs	2	15–20
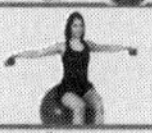	58	lateral raises	shoulders	2	20
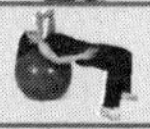	78	triceps extensions (back on ball)	triceps	2	20
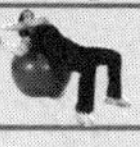	150	cross-body twists	obliques	2	15

slim and trim: level 2
three times a week for 20–30 minutes

With this three-times-a-week program, I've designed three individual workouts. Each of these slimming workouts incorporates upper- and lower-body work on each weight work day. Notice that you train your legs every time you work with weights, but you target different upper-body muscle groups from one workout to the next. Remember, the legs are the largest muscle group and when you work them, you burn more calories than when you work other muscle groups. For this reason, legs training better stimulates overall body-fat reduction; thus, it's included three times a week.

Changing exercises from one upper-body muscle group to another, from one weight session to the next, will also help you stimulate body fat burning more effectively than simply performing the same exercises each time you workout. Another technique that is helpful is to use heavier weights. As I mentioned in this program's introduction, you should aim to include heavier weights as your fitness level improves. Make a goal of completing one set of each exercise with level 4 weights. This set should be the last one for those exercises that necessitate using a weight.

WEEKLY SCHEDULE	
MONDAY	Workout 1
TUESDAY	20 min. cardio
WEDNESDAY	Workout 2
THURSDAY	20 min. cardio
FRIDAY	Workout 3
SATURDAY	20 min. cardio
SUNDAY	rest

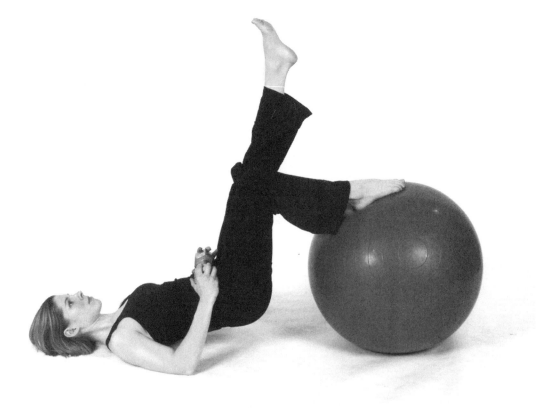

SLIM AND TRIM: LEVEL 2

workout 1

	PAGE	EXERCISE	TARGET	SETS	REPS
	128	wall squat curls	legs, biceps	3	20
	68	flat chest presses	chest	2	20
	74	incline chest flyes	chest	2	20
	56	triceps kickbacks (seated)	triceps	2	20
	142	abs crunches (feet on ball)	abs	1–2	15

workout 2

	PAGE	EXERCISE	TARGET	SETS	REPS
	120	back extensions	lower back, hamstrings, glutes	2	15–20
	122	reverse back extensions	lower back, glutes	2	15–20
	104	dumbbell rows (hand on ball)	back	2	20
	90	preacher curls	biceps	2	20
	152	side twists	abs, obliques	2	15

workout 3

	PAGE	EXERCISE	TARGET	SETS	REPS
	130	lunges	legs	2	15–20
	132	side lunges	inner & outer thighs	2	15–20
	60	shoulder presses	shoulders	2	20
	62	front raises (seated)	shoulders	2	20
	146	reverse crunches	lower abs	2	15

slim and trim: level 3
three times a week for 45 minutes

This ultimate fat-burning program puts you on the fast track to shedding body fat. If you can devote 30–45 minutes to exercise six days a week (three 45-minute weight sessions and three 30-minute cardio sessions), you can make phenomenal progress in reducing your body fat levels (coupled with a few simple tweaks to your nutrition program).

This program gives you three separate weight workouts that you should be able to complete in about 45 minutes each. Each workout should be performed once a week. You can build your week as you choose. Please see the sample schedules for two possibilities.

There are a couple of differences between this workout and the Level 2 workout. First, the Level 3 program starts with stretching moves on each weight training day. Stretching is an important component of overall fitness; I'd like to emphasize it at the other levels as well, but given the time constraint of

WEEK ONE	
MONDAY	Workout 1
TUESDAY	30 min. cardio
WEDNESDAY	Workout 2
THURSDAY	30 min. cardio
FRIDAY	Workout 3
SATURDAY	30 min. cardio
SUNDAY	rest

WEEK TWO	
MONDAY	30 min. cardio (a.m.) Workout 1 (p.m.)
TUESDAY	30 min. cardio
WEDNESDAY	Workout 2
THURSDAY	30 min. cardio
FRIDAY	Workout 3
SATURDAY	rest
SUNDAY	rest

those workouts, something had to give. If you have time, no matter your fitness level or goal, you should incorporate stretching as one of the best ways to combat the aging process. (See "Warming Up and Stretching," page 13.)

Second, this program asks you to perform more sets and more exercises. Now you will work individual body parts more fully during each session. Instead of performing only one exercise to target each body part, often you will perform two exercises consecutively for the same body part. This additional stimulation will encourage a little

more muscle growth and fat burning. Note that for the upper-body parts such as chest and triceps, you only work them once a week, doing all the work for each upper-body part during its respective workout. Another technique that is helpful is to use heavier weights. As I mentioned in this program's introduction, you should aim to include heavier weights as your fitness level improves. Make a goal of completing one to two sets of each exercise with level 4 weights. These sets should be the last ones for those exercises.

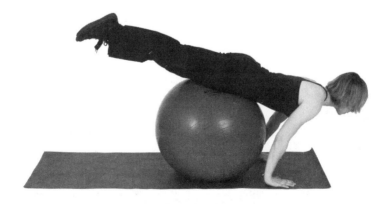

workout 1

	PAGE	EXERCISE	TARGET	SETS	REPS
	164	hip stretch	hips	1–2	1
	162	side stretch	abs, back	1–2	1
	128	wall squat curls	legs, biceps	4	20
	68	flat chest presses	chest	3	20
	74	incline chest flyes	chest	3	20
	54	triceps extensions (seated)	triceps	3	20
	140	abs crunches (back on ball)	abs	2	15

workout 2

	PAGE	EXERCISE	TARGET	SETS	REPS
	158	back bend stretch	back, abs	1–2	1
	160	spine stretch	back	1–2	1
	120	back extensions	lower back, hamstrings, glutes	2	15–20
	96	dumbbell rows (chest on ball)	back	3	20
	90	preacher curls	biceps	3	20
	52	hammer curls	biceps	3	20
	148	side crunches	obliques	2	15

workout 3

	PAGE	EXERCISE	TARGET	SETS	REPS
	164	hip stretch	hips	1–2	1
	166	roll-out stretch	shoulders, back	2–3	1
	130	lunges	legs	3	15–20
	134	lateral leg raises	thighs, glutes	3	15–20
	60	shoulder presses	shoulders	3	20
	58	lateral raises	shoulders	3	20
	146	reverse crunches	lower abs	2–3	15

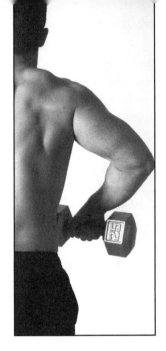

muscle bound

This program targets men and women who have a primary goal of enhancing their muscle mass. Typically, this is the goal of more men than women who start exercise programs, but I'd like to stress the advantages of this exercise goal for both sexes. The more muscle mass you have, the more calories your body needs each day just to maintain its body mass. The bottom line is that this allows you to eat more food without storing it as body fat. Once you have added muscle mass, it also encourages your body to use body fat as an energy source, as long as you're on a reasonable nutrition program, eating several smaller meals a day.

Often, women fear that they will get too muscular, but I contend that this is a false fear. It's important to realize that the natural hormone levels of the average female make it nearly impossible to become hugely muscular. When women first undergo a muscle-building program, they may, over the first few weeks, see a slight size increase in certain body parts. This is due to the rapid growth of muscle mass as the body quickly accommodates to training, and to the comparatively slow rate of body-fat reduction. Give it time (a couple months or

so) and you'll see that your body-fat levels begin to shrink and the amount of muscle you're building begins to plateau. The result is a much better balance of muscle mass and body fat. You'll have a little more build in the upper body, better shape in your legs, and a tighter, much more pleasing waistline. Ultimately, you'll have a thinner, better proportioned body. Your clothes will fit better, and you'll better like the way you look, both in and out of clothes. If you are one of the rare women who does get too muscular, you don't need to worry. One of the

easiest things in the world to do is to reduce muscle mass. Cutting back on the amount of weight-training exercise (sets, reps or weight) will rapidly allow you to reduce your total muscle mass.

Getting the most out of your workout

The workouts in this program are different from those in the previous two programs. To build muscle mass, you need to approach your training a little differently than when you're toning or trying to shed body fat. First, you need to stimulate

MUSCLE BOUND: INCREASING MUSCLE MASS		
	SCHEDULE	PROGRAM DESCRIPTION
LEVEL **1**	3 times a week; 30 min./session	For new or returning exercisers whose primary goal is to increase muscle mass.
LEVEL **2**	3 times a week; 45 min./session	For conditioned exercisers who want to work out three days a week to increase muscle mass.
LEVEL **3**	4 times a week; 45 min./session	For well-conditioned exercisers who want to commit to a full regimen designed to increase muscle mass.

individual muscle groups more intensely—you should work out with weights at least three times a week to reasonably expect to accomplish your goal of increasing muscle mass. Second, you target your body parts a little differently than you do when trying to firm up or shed body fat. You work each body part more exhaustively when you do train it, taking your muscles to "failure" (the level of fatigue where you cannot perform another rep without resting, struggling or breaking form). To do this, you work each body part only once a week, and then allow the rest of the week for that body part to recover and grow.

Muscles grow in the period after they are weight-trained, not during the exercise. Working them frequently (two or more times a week) can make them stronger and better toned, but to try to add muscle mass, you're better off working them fully once a week, then letting them recover. That's the core philosophy of the Muscle Bound program.

Reps and Weights

You want to use as much weight as you reasonably can and keep your reps a little lower than you do for the other training-goal strategies. Heavier weights performed for fewer reps is a much better muscle-building strategy than lighter weights with high reps. The rep requirements per set for this program are reduced from those in the other parts of the book. At first, this may seem odd, begging the question: *Shouldn't I do more work if I want to build more muscle mass?* The answer is "yes." But more work can be accomplished in ways other than by performing more reps.

Another key to muscle building is to use heavier weights and work with fewer reps. When you finish a set, your target muscles should be tired (often, with the other programs, your target muscles will feel more primed than exhausted). You should want to rest a bit before you're ready to do the next set. Ideally, your rest period should last 30 to 60 seconds before you perform the next set. For the Muscle Bound

program, however, you want to complete all the sets for one exercise before moving on to the next. (If you want to make the most of your rest time, you can incorporate some stretches or abs work). The objective is to stimulate your target muscle as much as you can in a relatively short period of time before stimulating it another way.

The sets listed in the workout charts are all working sets, meaning that if you want to perform a warm-up (I recommend including warm-up sets, especially with the first exercise for each body part), it doesn't count as one of your three working sets for that particular exercise. Again, warm-ups are good for pumping some blood into your target muscle group and helping you avoid injury. Interestingly, you'll find that as you accommodate to training, you feel stronger after performing a warm-up set than you do without one. For all these reasons, I recommend doing so.

As with the previous programs, I provide you with three levels of the Muscle Bound workout to allow you to determine the right place for you to begin.

Cardio Suggestions

For this Muscle Bound program, it's best to do your cardio on non-weights days. However, if your schedule doesn't allow this, go ahead and pair your weights and cardio days.

muscle bound: level 1
three times a week for 30 minutes

As noted in the introduction to this program, you should work out with weights at least three times a week to reasonably expect to add muscle mass. I also think that you need to work effectively for at least 30 minutes to maximize your results.

Therefore, the training demands of this lowest-level workout are significantly greater than the demands of the Level 1 workouts for the previous two programs. If you are just returning to exercise, or are a first-timer, you might consider following one of the other Level 1 workouts for four to six weeks (you can do them three times a week, though) before jumping into this program. This will prime your entire body for muscle building, as well as create the conditioning necessary for this program. Overall, you'll find you

get better, faster results by starting more slowly and working with your body than you will by jumping in over your head.

If you're already on an exercise program and would like to build more muscle mass, then Level 1 may be just right for you. Even if you've just been walking three times a week, you're probably ready to start with this program. If you have any doubts, however, perform two to three weeks of one of the other programs (Level 2 of the Slim and Trim program would be a good transition workout).

With this program, you'll note that each workout directly targets one or two different body parts each workout. Workout One focuses on legs and abs; Workout Two hits your chest and shoulders; while Workout Three targets back and arms.

WEEKLY SCHEDULE	
MONDAY	Workout 1
TUESDAY	20 min. cardio
WEDNESDAY	Workout 2
THURSDAY	20 min. cardio
FRIDAY	Workout 3
SATURDAY	20 min. cardio
SUNDAY	rest

Weight levels

If you are a beginner, you should use level 1 weights. If you have been training for a while, you can start with level 2 and 3 weights (depending on your fitness level). Try to progress to level 4 weights for most sets; as your conditioning and strength improve, you should begin to integrate some level 5 weights (as your last set for basic movements). See the chart on page 19 for an overview to the levels.

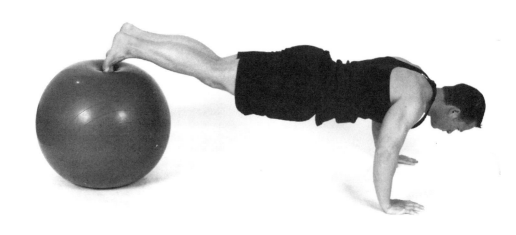

MUSCLE BOUND: LEVEL 1

workout 1

	PAGE	EXERCISE	TARGET	SETS	REPS
	128	wall squats	legs	3	15
	130	lunges	legs	3	10
	124	hamstrings curls	hamstrings	2	10
	132	side lunges	inner & outer thighs	2	8
	140	abs crunches (back on ball)	abs	2	15

workout 2

	PAGE	EXERCISE	TARGET	SETS	REPS
	70	incline chest presses	chest	2	10
	110	push-ups (feet on ball)	chest	2	10
	72	flat chest flyes	chest	2	10
	60	shoulder presses	shoulders	3	10
	58	lateral raises	shoulders	2	10

workout 3

	PAGE	EXERCISE	TARGET	SETS	REPS
	104	dumbbell rows (hand on ball)	back	3	10
	96	dumbbell rows (chest on ball)	back	2	10
	50	alternate biceps curls	biceps	2	10
	52	hammer curls	biceps	2	10
	154	hip raises	abs, glutes, hip flexors	2	15

muscle bound: level 2
three times a week for 45 minutes

Level 2 is an extension of Level 1, designed primarily for two groups: 1) Those who have achieved a fitness level that allows them to complete the training volume of a full 45-minute workout. 2) Those who have the time to do so.

The 45-minute workout is just about the best length of a workout for muscle building. Many hardcore enthusiasts weight train for an hour or an hour and a half or longer, but much of this is a waste of time, and even counterproductive. You can only stimulate your target muscle group so much in one workout to create the environment for ideal results. Training past this point can tear your muscle mass down, leading to days of soreness, and over time,

potentially to injury. Training with intensity for a moderate amount of time allows you to efficiently train your muscles and then get on with the other elements of your life.

These workouts are fairly demanding on your target muscles. To complete this workout in 45 minutes, you need to keep rest periods to about 60 seconds after each set. Again, perform all sets for one exercise before moving on to the next. This workout has you perform three sets of each exercise with a relatively heavy weight that still allows you to complete ten reps.

Weight levels
Since you have been training for a while, you can start with level 2 and 3 weights. Begin to

progress up to using level 4 weights for most sets. As your conditioning and strength improve, you should begin to integrate level 5 weights as your last set for basic movements for all weighted movements. See the chart on page 19 for an overview to the levels.

WEEKLY SCHEDULE	
MONDAY	Workout 1
TUESDAY	20–30 min. cardio
WEDNESDAY	Workout 2
THURSDAY	20–30 min. cardio
FRIDAY	Workout 3
SATURDAY	20–30 min. cardio
SUNDAY	rest

MUSCLE BOUND: LEVEL 2

workout 1

	PAGE	EXERCISE	TARGET	SETS	REPS
	128	wall squats	legs	3	10
	130	lunges (with weights)	legs	3	10
	134	lateral leg raises	thighs, glutes	3	10
	124	hamstrings curls	hamstrings	3	10
	136	seated calf raises	calves	3	10
	142	abs crunches (feet on ball)	abs	3	10

MUSCLE BOUND: LEVEL 2

workout 2

	PAGE	EXERCISE	TARGET	SETS	REPS
	104	dumbbell rows (hand on ball)	back	3	10
	76	pullovers	back	3	10
	114	walk-arounds (feet on ball)	whole body	3	1*
	64	shrugs	trapezius	3	10
	90	preacher curls	biceps	3	10
	80	inline curls	biceps	3	10

workout 3

	PAGE	EXERCISE	TARGET	SETS	REPS
	68	flat chest presses	chest	3	10
	74	incline chest flyes	chest	3	10
	60	shoulder presses	shoulders	3	10
	86	front raises (chest on ball)	shoulders	3	10
	54	triceps extensions (seated)	triceps	3	10
	116	triceps dips (with weight)	triceps	3	10

1 revolution in each direction

muscle bound: level 3
four times a week for 45 minutes

If you're truly serious about adding muscle mass and you have the fitness level to support it, then working out four times a week with weights for about 45 minutes is the best strategy. This workout takes the strategies of the other levels in this program and intensifies them somewhat. Workout One target legs and abs; Workout Two focuses on chest and triceps; Workout Three hits back and biceps; and Workout Four targets shoulders, traps, calves and abs. This is a full-body workout that you will complete once a week.

By increasing your training by one day a week, you are able to more effectively target each muscle group, giving it the ideal amount of stimulation for muscle growth. Note that biceps

and triceps are trained separately here, and that each is trained with a complementary muscle group (e.g., biceps with back, triceps with chest). This allows for even better recovery for these body parts, which is crucial since you'll be training them with a little more volume than at the lower levels of the Muscle Bound program. Training volume, as well as weight, is a great way to increase intensity, and thus muscular stimulation. Again, note that body parts are then given the rest of the week off for recovery.

Weight levels

Since you have been training consistently, you should begin this program with level 3 weights (feel free to use lighter

weights for warm-up sets, not included in the chart below). Begin to progress up to using level 4 weights for most sets. As your conditioning and strength improve, you should begin to integrate level 5 weights as your last set or two for basic movements for all weighted movements. See the chart on page 19 for an overview to the levels.

WEEKLY SCHEDULE	
MONDAY	Workout 1
TUESDAY	Workout 2
WEDNESDAY	20–30 min. cardio
THURSDAY	Workout 3
FRIDAY	Workout 4
SATURDAY	20–30 min. cardio
SUNDAY	rest

MUSCLE BOUND: LEVEL 3

workout 1

PAGE	EXERCISE	TARGET	SETS	REPS
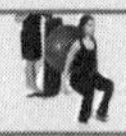 128	wall squats	legs	3	10
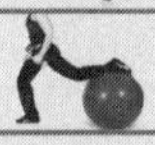 130	lunges (with weights)	legs	3	10
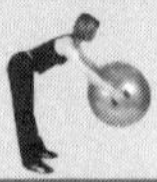 126	stiff-legged deadlifts	hamstrings, glutes lower back	3	10
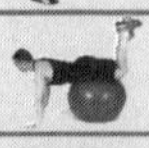 124	hamstrings curls	hamstrings	3	10
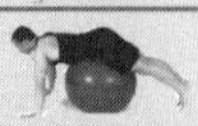 122	reverse back extensions	lower back, glutes	3	10
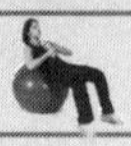 140	abs crunches (back on ball)	abs	3	10

MUSCLE BOUND: LEVEL 3

workout 2

PAGE	EXERCISE	TARGET	SETS	REPS
70	incline chest presses	chest	3	10
100	push-ups (hands on ball)	chest	3	10
72	flat chest flyes	chest	3	10
116	triceps dips	triceps	3	10
78	triceps extensions (back on ball)	triceps	3	10
56	triceps kickbacks (seated)	triceps	3	10

workout 3

PAGE	EXERCISE	TARGET	SETS	REPS
96	dumbbell rows (chest on ball)	back	3	10
76	pullovers	back	3	10
106	walk-arounds (hands on ball)	whole body	3	1*
50	alternate biceps curls	biceps	3	10
90	concentration curls	biceps	3	10
52	hammer curls	biceps	3	10
92	wrist curls	forearms	2	10

workout 4

PAGE	EXERCISE	TARGET	SETS	REPS
60	shoulder presses	shoulders	3	10
62	front raises (seated)	shoulders	3	10
84	rear delt flyes	shoulders	3	10
136	seated calf raises	calves	3	10
144	roll-up crunches	abs, obliques	3	10
64	shrugs	trapezius	3	10

*1 revolution in each direction

muscle bound 3

part three:
the exercises

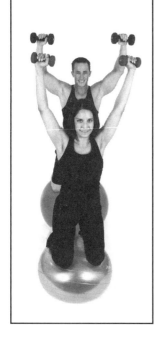

weights on the ball: time for action

This part of the book contains the nuts and bolts of the *Weights on the Ball* exercises so that you can implement the programs in Part Two. I've divided the exercises by your positioning on the ball, with the targeted body parts noted in the right-hand corner. In this section are thorough explanations of the positioning and performance of each exercise. Many elements of these exercises are obvious (such as putting your feet on the floor), but I want to provide as much information as I can for everyone who reads this book.

While some of the instruction is basic, some of it is quite subtle (such as the instruction in many exercises to retract your shoulders throughout the movement—easier said than done, as you'll learn!). The ability to perform every step the first time you attempt an exercise may be daunting—but don't let it be! Do as much as you can, as well as you can. Keep the book beside you and re-read the exercise descriptions frequently. As you progress, your ability to perform these exercises will also improve. Some of the more-subtle directions will begin to make more sense to you after you have more experience with the exercises and have mastered the basic elements.

In addition, you can begin to implement some of the various "challenges" that we've included for most of the exercises. Some of these aren't much more difficult than the basic exercise. Others are quite taxing. Interestingly, based on your body and its own strengths, you may find that some "challenges" are easier than some of the basics. It just goes to show you that while we're all pretty much the same, we're all a little bit different, too.

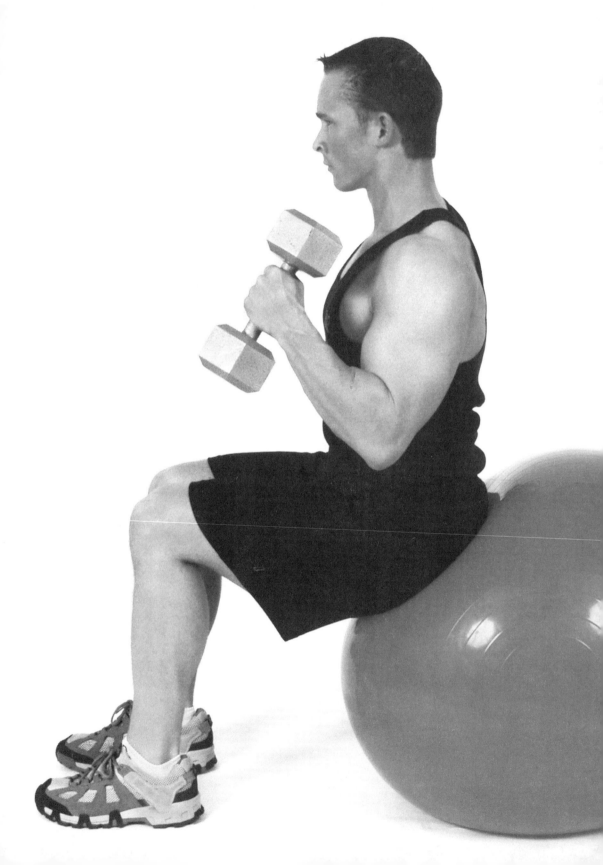

seat of power:
seated on the ball

This section provides you with detailed descriptions of some of the most basic weight exercises. By performing these upper-body exercises while seated on the ball, you are also helping to strengthen the core of your body while you target particular muscle groups such as biceps, triceps, shoulders or trapezius. Performing exercises in this seated position is an excellent way for beginners or those who have not exercised for a long time to adapt to working with weights and the ball, and the unique demands they place upon the body. As you progress, you'll also find that these are also excellent moves for intermediate and advanced exercises as well.

alternate biceps curls

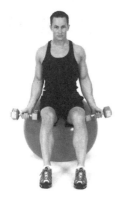

This is a basic exercise for building or toning the biceps, which lie along the front portion of your upper arms.

STARTING POSITION: Sit on the ball with a dumbbell in each hand, with your upper arms down by your sides and your palms facing out. Place both feet squarely on the floor and tighten your core muscles. Hold these tight throughout the movement.

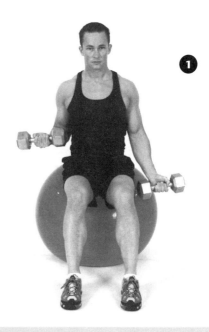

1

1 Keeping your upper arms perpendicular to the ground, curl one arm up toward your shoulder so that at the top of the move, your palm faces your shoulder.

variations

BASIC/INTERMEDIATE

Begin to curl with the second arm as you reach the top of the movement with the first. This will keep both arms in motion throughout the entire set, rather than allowing one arm to rest while you work the other. This strategy of continuous movement increases the intensity and demands on your target muscle.

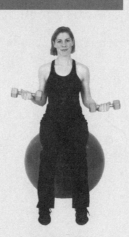

INTERMEDIATE

Raise one foot off the ground for the first half of the set, then switch and raise the other foot for the second half of the set.

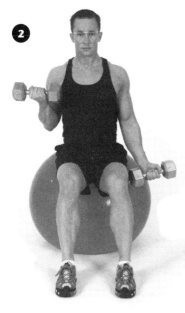

2 Squeeze your biceps at the top of the movement and hold for a second or two.

TIP

- Hold your biceps tight through the entire range of motion—don't allow them to relax as you lower the weight as this undercuts the effectiveness of the exercise.
- At the start of the movement, your palms can face one another, but twist your wrists as you lift the weights so that your palms face your shoulders.

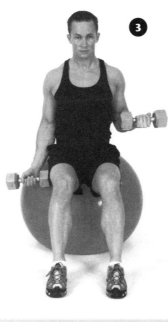

3 Lower the weight, feeling the stretch in your biceps. Switch directly to your other arm. Alternate until you complete your set.

INTERMEDIATE/ADVANCED

Perform this move while balanced on your knees on the ball. You may alternate or use both arms at the same time.

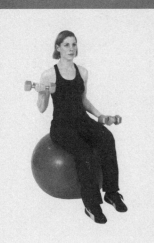

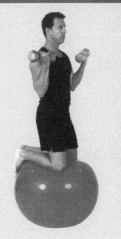

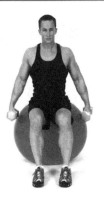

This movement targets your biceps and the brachialis, the small muscle between your triceps and biceps.

STARTING POSITION: Sit on the ball with a dumbbell in each hand. Let your arms hang at your sides with the palms facing inward. If the ball is at all in the way, extend your arms out to the side a little, away from your body. Place both feet squarely on the floor and tighten your core muscles, holding these tight throughout the exercise.

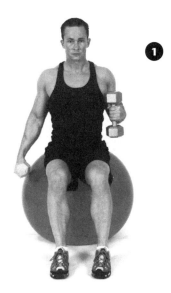

①

1 Without rotating your wrists or moving your upper arms, bring the dumbbell up until its upper head is close to your shoulder.

variations

BASIC/INTERMEDIATE

Begin to curl with the second arm as you reach the top of the movement with the first. This will keep both arms in motion throughout the entire set, rather than allowing one arm to rest while you work the other. This strategy of continuous movement increases the intensity and demands on your target muscle.

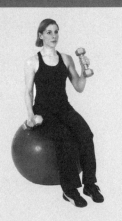

INTERMEDIATE

Raise one foot off the ground for the first half of the set, then switch and raise the other foot for the second half of the set.

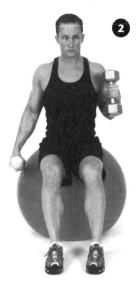

2 Squeeze your upper arm at the top of the movement.

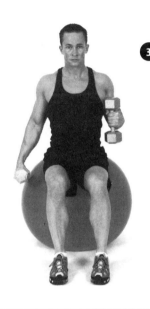

3 Holding that contraction, stretch the muscles in your upper arm as you slowly lower the weight back to the starting position. Repeat on the other side.

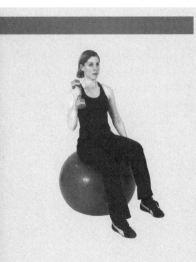

ADVANCED

Perform this move balanced on your knees on the ball. You may alternate or use both arms at the same time.

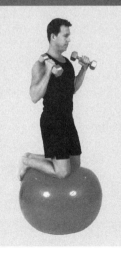

triceps extensions

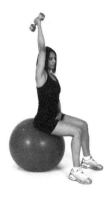

This triceps movement is an excellent exercise for adding definition to your triceps as it gives this muscle a nice stretch.

STARTING POSITION: Seated on the ball, raise a dumbbell up toward the ceiling; extend your arm fully but avoid locking your elbow. Place both feet squarely on the floor and tighten your core muscles. This is particularly important for an overhead movement, where the weight can have more effect on your balance. Maintain this tight posture throughout the movement.

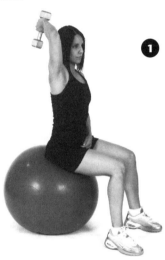

1

1 Keeping your upper arm stationary, bend your arm at the elbow. Lower the weight behind your head slowly and with control, feeling the stretch in your triceps. Take the weight as low as is comfortable.

variations

BASIC/INTERMEDIATE

Perform reps with both arms at the same time. This requires much more balance and core tightening, and you will lose the ability to spot or support yourself.

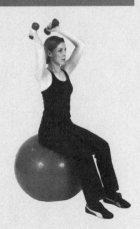

INTERMEDIATE

Performing reps with both arms at the same time, raise one foot off the ground. Perform reps slowly to take advantage of the effect this has on your core.

2

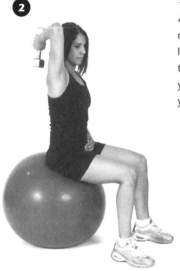

2 Raise the weight, activating from the center of your triceps muscle rather than using the leverage of your elbow joint. At the top of the movement, extend your arm fully but avoid locking your elbow.

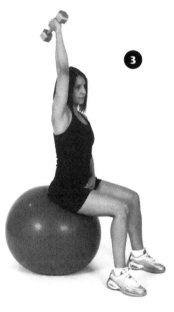

3

3 Contract your triceps, hold for a second and begin your next rep. Complete all reps for one side, then switch and perform with the other arm.

TIP

- You can use your second hand to support the working arm in one of two ways: 1) Hold your upper arm, helping to keep it from moving. 2) Spot yourself by gently assisting your working arm by pressing on your forearm as you extend the weight upward.
- The dumbbell can angle back across your body or straight back, depending on the natural flexibility of your shoulder complex; most people should stop with their lower arm just about parallel to the ground.

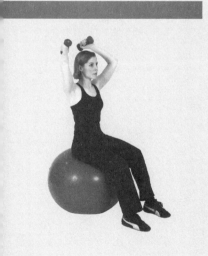

ADVANCED

Perform this move balanced on your knees on the ball.

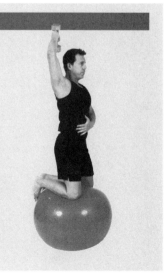

triceps kickbacks

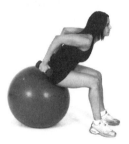

This is a great exercise to help bring out the "horseshoe" of the triceps—that indentation at the back of the arm that both men and women covet.

STARTING POSITION: Seated on the ball, bend forward at the waist, keeping your spine in its neutral position. Widen your foot placement as necessary to make this possible. Holding a dumbbell in each hand, extend your upper arms behind you so that they are parallel to the ground. Your elbows should be bent at about a 90-degree angle, the weights hanging at your sides with palms facing inward.

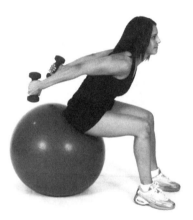

1 Extend the weights back until your arms are straight behind you and about parallel to the ground.

variations

BASIC/INTERMEDIATE

Perform your reps one arm at a time. You can alternate arms, or perform a full set with one arm then do the other. This variety will challenge your balance a little more than the two-arm variety.

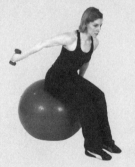

INTERMEDIATE

Bring your feet closer together and lift one off the ground. Do so without compromising your lower-back positioning. Perform either the one- or two-arm version.

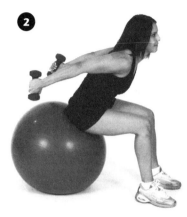

2 At full extension, squeeze the backs of your arms, envisioning the development of the horseshoe. Hold that for one second.

3 Keeping the tension in your upper arm, stretch your triceps as you bring the weight back. You can stop when your lower arms are perpendicular to the ground, or continue farther until the weights begin to rise toward your armpits. This provides a greater stretch but encourages you to swing the weight—try to avoid swinging.

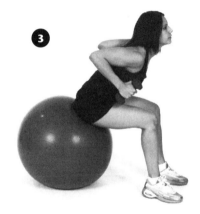

ADVANCED

Perform this move while balanced on your knees on the ball.

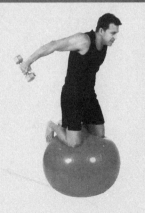

lateral raises

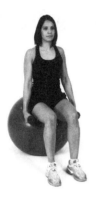

Performed correctly, lateral raises are an excellent exercise for adding detail to the outside of your shoulder. By creating a broader look through the shoulder, you provide a slimming effect on your midsection. This exercise targets all three heads of the deltoids, particularly the middle one.

STARTING POSITION: Seated on the ball, hold a weight in each hand with your palms facing one another. Allow the weights to hang at your sides, or hold them just above where they would otherwise touch the balance ball. You should keep a slight bend at your elbows and maintain this angle throughout the entire set. Rotate your shoulders back and keep your spine in its neutral position. Maintain your posture and keep your entire upper body in one plane throughout this exercise.

1

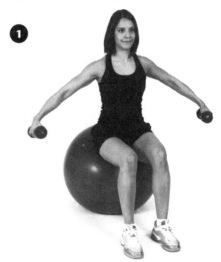

1 Raise the weights out to your sides, using the muscles at the sides of your shoulders, until your arms are parallel to the ground with your palms facing downward.

variations

BASIC/INTERMEDIATE

Perform the exercise one arm at a time. Complete all reps for one arm, then switch to the other. This asymmetrical movement requires more stabilization.

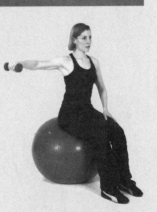

INTERMEDIATE

Perform the exercise with one foot off the ground.

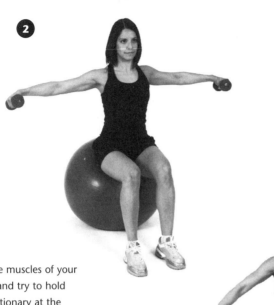

2

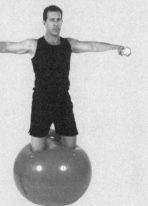

3

2 Squeeze the muscles of your
shoulders, and try to hold
the weights stationary at the
top of the movement for a second
or two.

3 Begin to slowly lower the
weight, fighting gravity with
the muscles of your shoulders.
Stop before your hands or the
weights come in contact with
the ball.

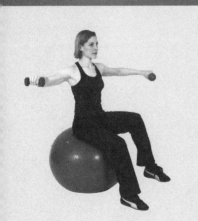

ADVANCED

Perform this move while
balanced on your knees on
the ball.

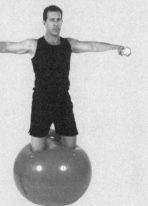

shoulder presses

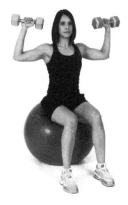

Dumbbell shoulder presses are one of the best overall shoulder developers, targeting the whole shoulder complex. Heavier weights allow you to build more shoulder mass, while lighter weights improve your overall shape and body symmetry.

STARTING POSITION: Sit on the ball with a dumbbell in each hand. Hold the weights close to your shoulders with your palms facing forward. Raise your arms so that your elbows are out to the sides and at shoulder height or just slightly below. Move your hands out to the side until they are directly above your elbows; your lower arms should be perpendicular to the ground. Hold your abdominals tight and keep your spine in its neutral position.

variations

INTERMEDIATE

Lift one foot off the ground, keeping your abs as tight as you can. This variation is more challenging for this exercise than for others while seated on the ball because it's an overhead movement.

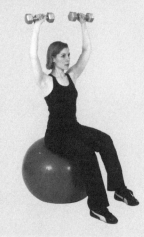

INTERMEDIATE/ADVANCED

Hold your raised leg parallel to the ground as you press the weight overhead, making certain to keep your spine in the neutral position and your abs tight.

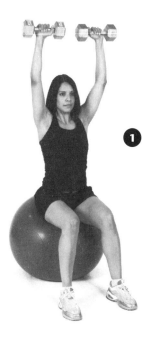

1 Smoothly press the weights up over your head. Extend your arms fully but avoid locking your elbows, keeping the weight under control with the power in your shoulders. At the top, the weights can come close together but should not touch one another. Contract the muscles in your shoulders at the top of the movement.

TIP

• Avoid allowing your abs to relax at any time during the set. Overhead movements on the ball require a substantial amount of stabilization from your core. Holding your abs tight helps you maintain your balance.

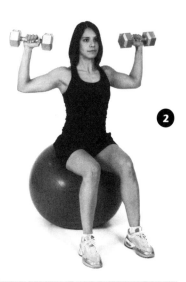

2 Lower the weights slowly, feeling the stretch in your shoulders.

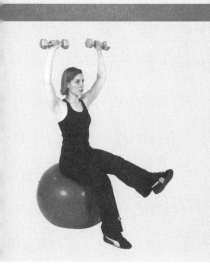

ADVANCED

Perform this exercise while balanced on your knees on the ball.

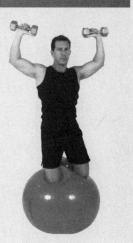

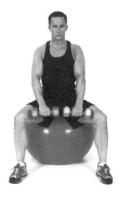

This exercise also targets the shoulder complex, but more directly works the front deltoids. Front raises are a great detail enhancer, and many people are proportionally weaker in the front deltoids than they are in the middle deltoids.

STARTING POSITION: Sit on the ball with your legs wide apart—more than shoulder width—to allow you to hold both dumbbells between your legs, with the palms facing the ball. You should have a slight bend in your elbows; maintain that bend throughout the entire set. Tighten your abs and hold your spine in its neutral position throughout the movement. Carefully maintain your stability (you don't want momentum to pitch you backwards off the ball!).

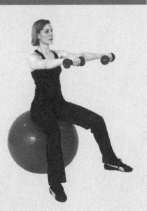

1 Deliberately raise one weight out in front of you until your arm is parallel to the ground with your palm facing downward.

variations

BASIC/INTERMEDIATE

Raise both weights at the same time. This requires a little more stabilization, so make certain that your abs are tight. It also reduces rest time between reps, forcing your deltoids to work harder in a shorter space of time.

INTERMEDIATE/ADVANCED

If your balance is good, you can try to raise one foot off the ground while raising the weights. Place a dumbbell on each side of your leg for stability since this move is kind of tricky; you might also attempt it with a much lighter weight at first.

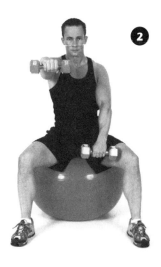

2 At the top of the movement, squeeze your front delt, along the top of your arm near your chest. Hold for a second.

TIP

- Make sure that your shoulders are rotated back throughout this movement. There's a tendency to allow the weight to pull your shoulders forward. Fight it! When your shoulder travels forward, it activates your trapezius. This can undercut the effectiveness of the exercise and potentially lead to injury.

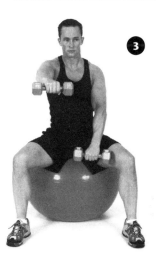

3 Maintaining that tension in your front deltoid, slowly lower the weight, fighting gravity with the strength of that target muscle. Stop just before the weight touches the ball. Alternate with the other arm.

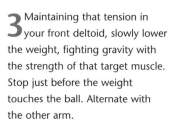

ADVANCED

Perform this exercise while balanced on your knees on the ball.

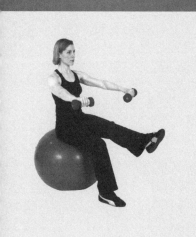

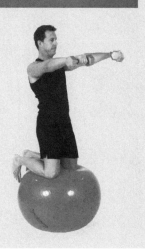

shrugs

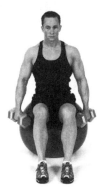

Shrugs develop your trapezius muscle, the large butterfly-shaped muscle that runs across your shoulders at the base of your neck and down into the center of your back. It's also a good exercise for relieving a tight neck from repetitive-motion activities such as working at a computer.

STARTING POSITION: Sit on the ball with your feet about shoulder width apart (but close enough together that your legs don't otherwise get in the way of the movement). Hold a dumbbell in each hand at your side with your palms facing inward. Avoid letting the weights touch the ball; you can bend your elbows slightly or hold the weights angled out a little to the sides to prevent this. Maintain the bend in your elbows throughout the movement.

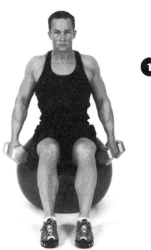

1

1 Lift your shoulders up and back. Squeeze your trapezius as you raise your shoulders—think about contracting the center of your back as well as the upper traps along your shoulders.

variations

INTERMEDIATE

Perform shrugs with one foot off the ground, switching feet midway through your set.

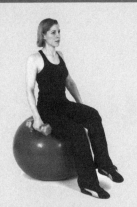

INTERMEDIATE/ADVANCED

Extend your foot out in front of you so that your leg is parallel to the ground. Maintain a neutral spinal position as you do this.

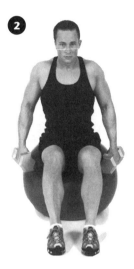

2 At the top of the movement, hold and contract.

TIP

- Focus on both the center of your back and the upper traps to develop the entire muscle.
- For best results, emphasize strict form with a forced contraction instead of using heavier weights.

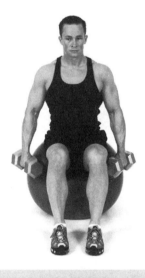

3

3 Still holding your trapezius taut, lower the weights back to the start position.

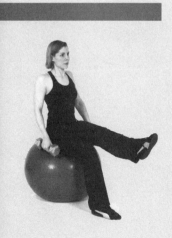

ADVANCED

Perform this move while balanced on your knees on the ball.

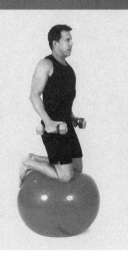

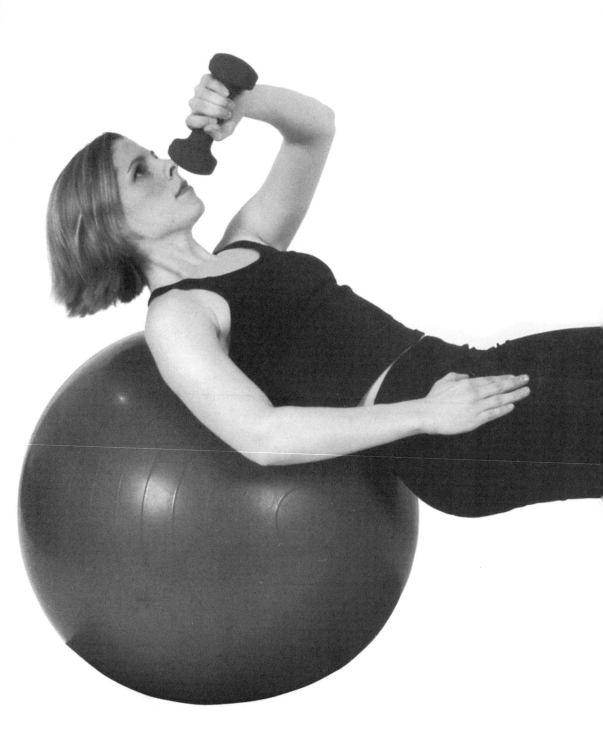

back to basics:
back on the ball

After the seated position, the next most basic position is probably placing your back against the ball. This position allows you to target several upper-body muscles groups such as chest, triceps, back and biceps. In addition, see the section on abs for more back-on-the-ball moves. One of the advantages of performing these moves on the ball rather than on a solid surface such as a weight bench is that you also work the stabilizers that support these larger muscle groups. This work will strengthen not only the larger muscles but the stabilizers as well, which has the benefit of more fully and naturally developing your entire body.

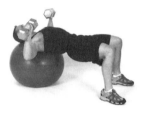

Chest presses can be either a great muscle builder or a toner, depending on the amount of weight you use and the number of repetitions you perform.

STARTING POSITION: Holding two dumbbells, sit on the ball and move your feet forward. Roll the ball beneath you until it is aligned under your upper back; your head should touch the ball, if possible, for additional support. Raise your hips so that your body is essentially in one plane from your knees to the top of your head. Place your feet square so that your knees are directly above your ankles. Position your legs with your knees comfortably apart for ideal stabilization. Hold the weights so that they are resting near your armpits at the start of the movement.

1

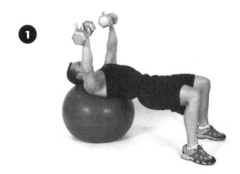

1 Keeping your forearms perpendicular to the ground, press the weight up until your arms are fully extended but do not lock your elbows. Keep your shoulders back as you press up so that your chest does the work.

variations

BASIC

At the top of the movement, give your pecs an additional squeeze, still keeping your shoulders back. Hold that contraction for a couple of seconds. This will intensify the work of your pectorals.

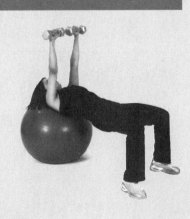

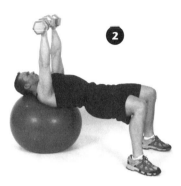

2 At the top of the movement, squeeze your pectorals. The weights should be a little closer than shoulder width apart, but avoid clanging them together.

TIP

- Notice how the ball helps you open up your chest when you support yourself with the outer portion of your shoulder blades rather than with the middle of your back. This can help you stimulate your pectorals even more effectively, and also helps you retract your shoulders.

- You don't want to lock your elbows at the top of the press because this takes the stress off your chest muscles and allows them to relax, preventing them from working as intensely as they should.

3 With your shoulders still retracted, lower the dumbbells smoothly and at a moderately slow pace to prevent gravity from doing the work for you. As you do this, feel that stretch across your chest—that's the sign that the exercise is working. Without resting unless absolutely necessary, begin your next rep.

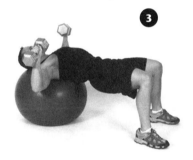

INTERMEDIATE

Try raising one foot off the ground while performing this exercise. This will recruit more of your core, helping to strengthen your body overall. Do this with a lighter weight because this is more of a toning-style variation.

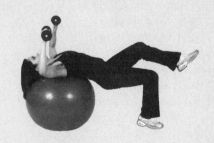

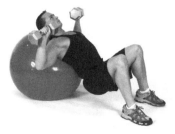

While similar to the flat chest press, this movement targets the upper pectorals slightly more than the flat version does.

STARTING POSITION: Place your upper back on the ball, stabilizing with your feet about shoulder width apart, knees bent. Drop your hips as close to the ground as possible without losing the ball. You can arch your back slightly to open up your chest a bit. Hold a weight in each hand at your armpits with your palms facing your feet. Extend your head so that your upper spine maintains its natural curvature throughout the entire movement.

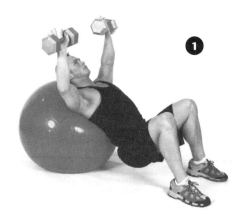

1 Using the power of your pectorals, press the weights up toward the ceiling. They can travel in a slight arc so that the weights are closer together at the top of the movement.

BASIC

At the top of the movement, give your pecs an additional squeeze, still keeping your shoulders back. Hold that contraction for a couple of seconds. This will intensify the work of your pectorals.

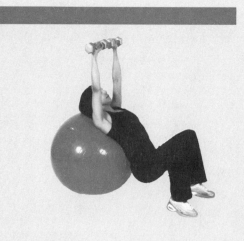

variations

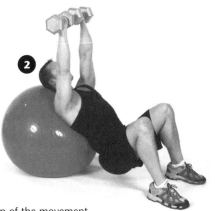

2

TIP

- Keep your shoulders retracted (rotated back toward the ground) throughout the set. There's a tendency to allow your shoulder joint to move forward as you press the weight up. This over-works the rear delts and traps, and undercuts the development of your target muscles.

2 At the top of the movement, your palms should be facing your feet and your arms should be straight, although avoid locking your elbows. Squeeze your pectorals.

3 Continuing to use your pecs, slowly lower the weight. Avoid letting gravity bring the weight back down with little effort on your part. At the bottom, feel the stretch in your pectorals, then begin the next rep.

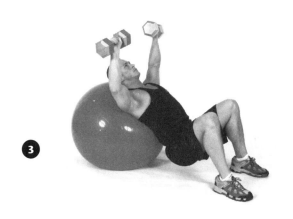

3

INTERMEDIATE

Try raising one foot off the ground while performing this exercise. This will recruit more of your core, helping to strengthen your body overall. Do this with a lighter weight because this is more of a toning-style variation.

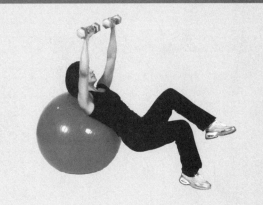

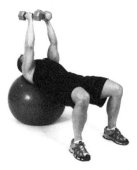

The pectoral muscles perform two functions: pressing away from the body and bringing your arms across your body. Flye movements fulfill this secondary function, important for balanced development of the upper body.

STARTING POSITION: Lie on the ball, balancing comfortably on the middle of your back. Allow your hips to drop only slightly lower than your knees, and space your feet about shoulder width apart so that you feel well stabilized. With a weight in each, extend your arms straight up toward the ceiling with your palms facing one another and a slight break at your elbows. Throughout, hold your head in its neutral position and maintain that break in your elbows.

1 Moving only from your shoulder joint, slowly lower the weights straight out to the side until your upper arms are parallel to the ground. If you are flexible, you can let your elbows dip slightly lower than your shoulders.

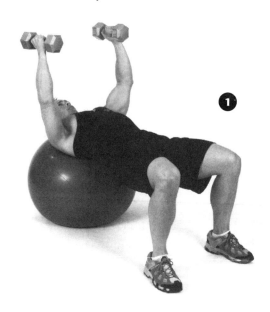

1

INTERMEDIATE

Perform this movement with one foot on the ground, knee bent, and the other raised.

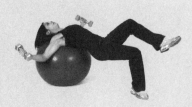

variations

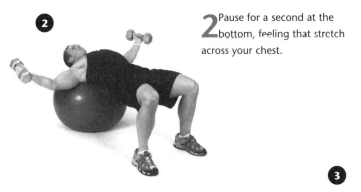

2 Pause for a second at the bottom, feeling that stretch across your chest.

TIP

- Keep your shoulders retracted (pulled back toward the ground) throughout the movement. When you press your shoulders forward, this activates your rear delts and traps, undercutting the workload on your pectorals.
- Contract your abdominals for further stabilization.
- Feel free to use a mat to help stabilize your feet.

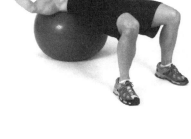

3 Pulling from your chest, begin to raise your arms back up to the start position.

4 Stop just short of allowing the weights to touch one another and squeeze your pectorals for a second before beginning the next rep.

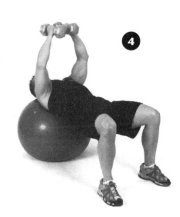

INTERMEDIATE/ADVANCED

To deepen the challenge, place the leg that touches the ground farther from your body and raise the other so that it is parallel to the ground.

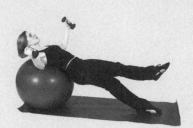

incline chest flyes

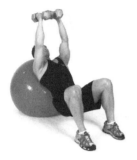

This movement is essentially the same as the flat chest flye, except the positioning shifts the emphasis to your upper chest.

STARTING POSITION: Place your upper back on the ball, stabilizing with your feet about shoulder width apart. Drop your hips as close to the ground as possible without losing the ball. You can arch your back slightly to open up your chest a bit. With a weight in each, extend your arms straight up toward the ceiling with your palms facing one another and a slight break at your elbows.

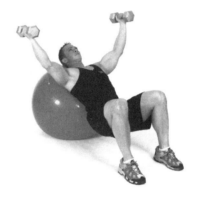

1

1 Moving only from the shoulder joint, slowly lower the weights straight out to the side until your upper arms are parallel to the ground. If you're flexible, you can take your elbows slightly lower than your shoulders.

variations

BASIC/INTERMEDIATE

Straighten your legs, and using only your heels for balance, perform this exercise.

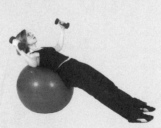

INTERMEDIATE

Perform this movement with one foot on the ground, knee bent, and the other raised.

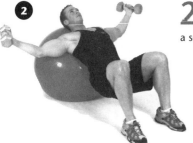

2 Feel and hold the stretch across your upper chest for a second.

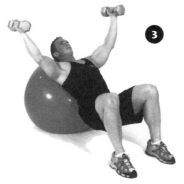

3 Activating your upper pectorals, pull the weights back up, maintaining the break at your elbows. Concentrate on the feeling in your chest.

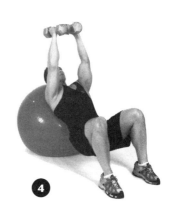

4 As you reach the top of the movement, squeeze your pectorals and hold that contraction for a second or two.

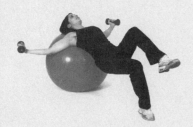

ADVANCED

To deepen the challenge, hold the leg that touches the ground straight and raise the other so that it's parallel to the ground.

pullovers

This upper-body movement can be useful in helping you develop both your chest and your back.

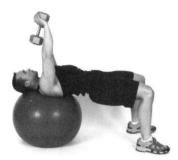

STARTING POSITION: Lie with your upper back comfortably on the middle of the ball so that your neck is also supported. Place your feet shoulder width apart out in front of you and raise your hips so that your body forms a line from your knees to the top of your head. Maintain your head and neck in this neutral position throughout the movement. With both hands, hold one dumbbell, aimed toward the ceiling, on your chest. Grasp the dumbbell by the upper head with your palms facing up toward the ceiling. Push the weight up until your arms are extended with only a slight break at your elbows. Maintain this elbow angle throughout the entire set.

1 Moving only your shoulder joints, slowly arc the weight overhead. Allow it to travel overhead toward the ground. Maintain strict control of the weight so that it doesn't simply fall.

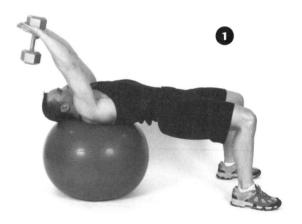

BASIC/INTERMEDIATE

Straighten your legs, place your feet together and, using only your heels for balance, perform this exercise.

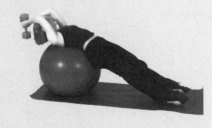

variations

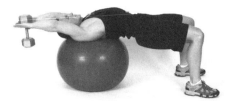

2

TIP

- For best results, contract the body part that you are trying to work and squeeze it. It may take a few sessions before you start differentiating between your pecs and back, but concentrating on your target muscle will help you emphasize that over the other.
- Hold your abdominals tight for further stabilization.
- Keep your shoulder rotated back toward the ground throughout the movement.

3

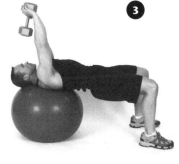

2 Take the weight to the point where your body forms one straight line from your knees to your extended arms. If this is challenging or painful, stop short of this position.

3 Pulling with your target muscle (chest or back), raise the weight back up until your arms are perpendicular to the ground.

4

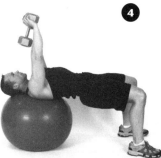

4 At the end of the rep, squeeze your target muscle (chest or back).

ADVANCED

To deepen the challenge, hold the leg that touches the ground straight and raise the other so that it is parallel to the ground.

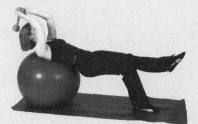

triceps extensions

This is a great exercise to target the triceps and add detail. It's also ideal for those who may have trouble with overhead versions due to shoulder injuries or limited flexibility.

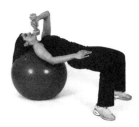

STARTING POSITION: Lying with your upper back on the ball, stabilize yourself with a shoulder-width stance. Lift your hips so that your body forms one line from your knees to the top of your head. With one hand, hold a dumbbell aimed upward against your upper chest or opposite shoulder, whichever feels more natural and allows you to feel your triceps working the most. The outside of your hand can contact the upper head of the dumbbell for support. Your upper arm should be perpendicular to the ground with your elbow bent at about a 90-degree angle. Hold the weight slightly off your chest and keep your upper arm stationary throughout the entire movement.

1 Using the power of your triceps, extend your lower arm upwards until it is aligned with your upper arm, perpendicular to the ground.

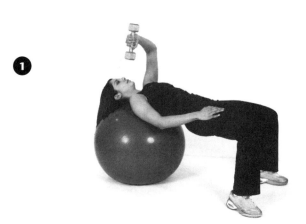

variations

BASIC

Perform this exercise with two arms overhead.

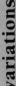

INTERMEDIATE

For more of a challenge, perform this movement with one foot on the ground, knee bent, and the other raised. You can do this one-arm cross-body, or two arms overhead.

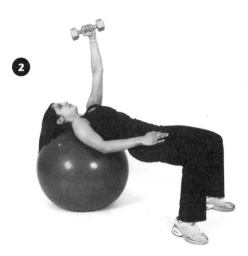

②

2 Squeeze your triceps at the peak of the movement.

3 Use your triceps rather than your elbow joint to lower the weight. Feel the stretch along the outside of that muscle.

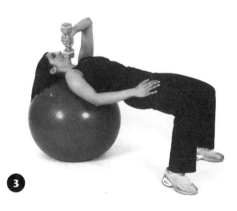

③

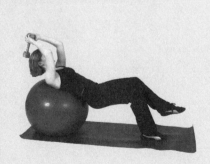

INTERMEDIATE/ADVANCED

To further increase the challenge, straighten your lifted leg and hold it parallel to the ground. You can do this one-arm cross-body, or two arms overhead.

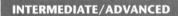

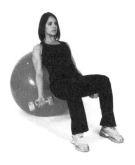

This is a great isolation movement for your biceps, particularly emphasizing the top portion near your shoulder joint.

STARTING POSITION: With your upper back on the ball, scootch forward, dropping your hips as close to the ground as possible without losing the ball. Your body, from your butt to the top of your head, should form a straight line that makes about a 45-degree angle with the ground. Avoid bending your head forward or backward to shift the muscle recruitment. Keep your spine in its neutral alignment up through your neck. Hold a dumbbell in each hand and allow your arms to hang nearly straight down. Open your chest just a bit so that your arms are slightly angled out from your body. If your upper arms contact the ball, though, that's fine.

1 Lift the weights up until your lower arms are nearly perpendicular to the ground. As you curl the weights up, the weights will travel in closer to your body.

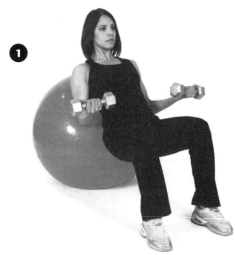

❶

variations

BASIC/INTERMEDIATE

To step it up a notch, you can perform this movement by alternating arms. This requires a little more stability work.

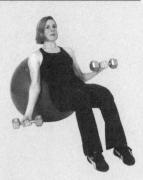

INTERMEDIATE

Keeping your knees bent, place your feet six inches to one foot farther away from the ball. This will force you to use more abdominal stabilization as you curl the weight.

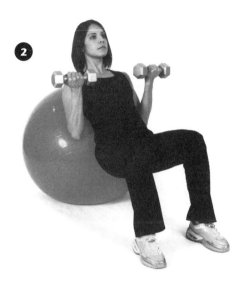

2

TIP

• Avoid moving your upper arms as you curl up; pull the weight with the power of your biceps.

• This is a more challenging movement than biceps curls seated on the ball (see page 50) so you should use slightly less weight (or use more weight for the seated variety).

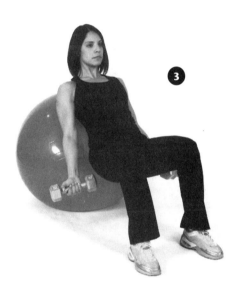

3

2 Squeeze your biceps at the top of the movement.

3 Lower the weight, feeling the stretch along the tops of your biceps.

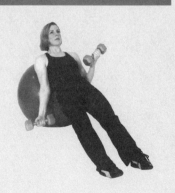

INTERMEDIATE/ADVANCED

Raise one foot off the ground and hold it out in front of you (you can bend your knee since this is an awkward position). Switch feet midway through the set.

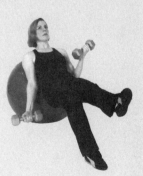

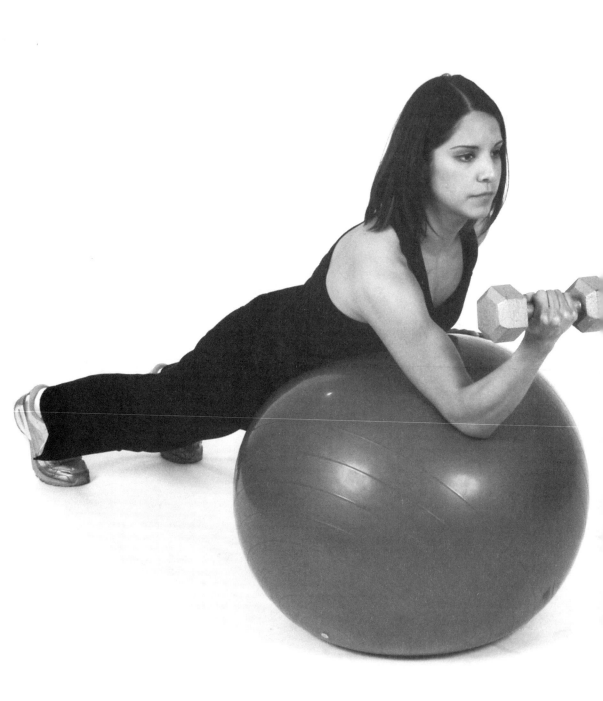

keeping up a good front: chest on the ball

These movements, where you lie face down with your chest pressed into the ball, can be slightly more difficult in terms of position than those where you sit or place your back against the ball. Nevertheless, many of these movements are basic weight-training movements, crucial for the overall development of your body. The exercises in this section target your shoulders, biceps, forearms and back while also requiring you to use more stabilizers both in the target area and in the core of your body.

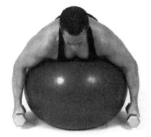

Rear delts are among the most difficult muscles of the body to isolate and define. The support of the ball can help you learn to feel the muscle working. Developing rear delts is not only important aesthetically, but can also benefit your posture and shoulder positioning during activities with repetitive movements such as working on a computer.

STARTING POSITION: From standing, place your lower chest on the ball so that you are facing downward with your feet shoulder-width behind you. Balance on your toes, forming a slight incline from feet to head. Hold a dumbbell in each hand and down to the side with your palms facing inward at shoulder width or slightly wider so as not to touch the ball. You can keep a slight, 10-degree bend at your elbows through the whole set. Hold your shoulders back and chest out throughout the movement.

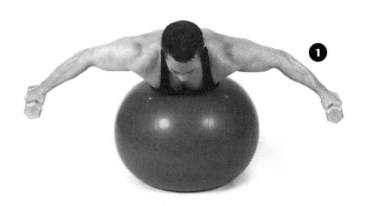

1 Moving your arms only from the shoulder joint, lift the weights up and out to the side. Raise your upper arms until they are parallel to the ground.

variations

BASIC

To make the exercise less strenuous, you can lower your knees to the ground. You can bend at the waist, but keep your spine in its neutral position.

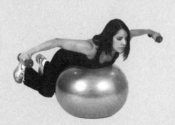

INTERMEDIATE

Hold one leg off the ground and extend it behind you (bonus points for pointing your toes!). This position will also allow your body to become more parallel to the ground, increasing your ability to target your rear delts in addition to requiring more stabilization of your body.

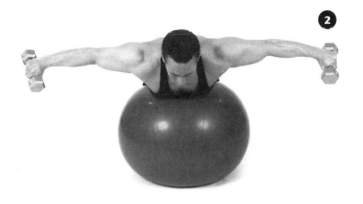

2

TIP

- The more parallel your body is to the ground, the easier it is to target your rear delts.

- Use a very light weight at first until you learn to isolate and contract your rear delts. Using too much weight forces you to recruit your traps and back muscles, making this a much less effective exercise for developing your rear delts.

- Avoid allowing your traps (the muscles in the middle of your back and at the base of your neck) to pinch together.

2 At the top of the movement, tense the muscles just at the back of your shoulders. Hold that contraction.

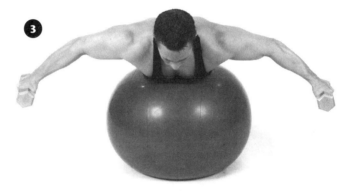

3

3 Lower the weights slowly without dropping your shoulders, making sure to concentrate on that target muscle. Stop before you contact the ball or your arms reach the perpendicular resting position. Move directly into the next rep.

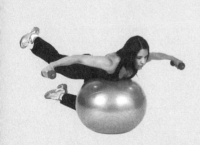

ADVANCED

Place your feet on a bench so that your entire body is one plane and parallel to the ground. This will force you to stabilize your core and better target your rear deltoids. Execute the exercise carefully and smoothly to avoid losing your balance.

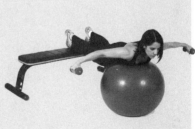

front raises

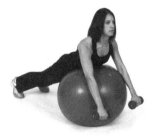

This movement develops the shoulders, particularly targeting the front delts. It's also much more challenging than front raises performed while seated on the ball (see page 62). This version allows for a greater range of motion, forcing your body to work from a mechanical disadvantage (often a positive when trying to develop muscle shape or mass).

STARTING POSITION: Stand in front of the ball and place your chest against it. Place your feet at shoulder width and maintain your balance from your toes. With the ball supporting your body at the lower part of your chest, take a weight in each hand with your arms hanging straight down in front of the ball, palms facing the ball.

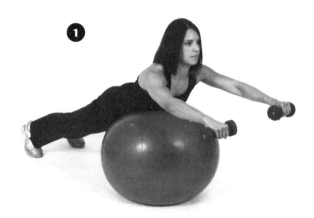

1 With straight arms, raise both weights slowly and with control out in front of you until they are parallel or slightly above parallel to the ground.

variations

BASIC

If holding a straight line from feet to head is too difficult, perform the exercise with your knees resting on the ground. You can bend at the waist, but keep your spine in its neutral position throughout.

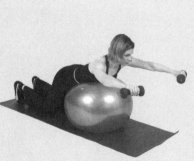

INTERMEDIATE

Bring your feet close together as you perform the movement. This forces you to stabilize more to avoid rocking from side to side.

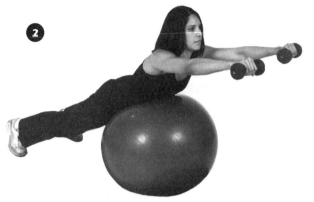

2

2 At the peak position, ideally, your body should make one line from your feet to your hands. At the top of the movement, squeeze your deltoids and hold for a second or two.

3 Keeping the action in your deltoids, slowly lower the weights as perpendicular to the ground as you can without allowing the weights or your arms to contact the ball. Move directly into the next rep.

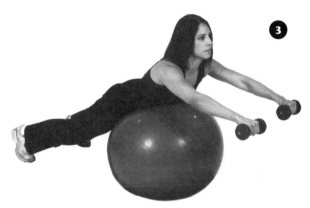

3

INTERMEDIATE/ADVANCED

Try lifting one leg behind you so that it is parallel to the ground.

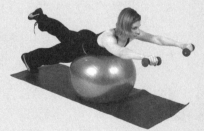

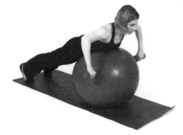

Shoulder rotation moves are often performed by those who have had shoulder injuries to promote rehabilitation. They're also excellent as a warm up and as a preventative for potential shoulder injuries. We recommend that weight trainers of all age and skill level incorporate them for this reason.

STARTING POSITION: From standing, place your lower chest on the ball so that you are facing downward with your feet shoulder width behind you. Balance on your toes, forming a slight incline from feet to head. Hold a dumbbell in each hand. Raise your elbows up and straight out to the sides of your shoulders so that your elbows and shoulders are all in one line, running parallel to the ground. Allow your lower arms to hang down perpendicular to the ground; your palms should face toward your feet. Throughout the set, keep your upper arms parallel to the ground and maintain your neck in its neutral position—don't allow your head to drop.

variations

INTERMEDIATE

Use slightly more weight but maintain controlled form. While this is not a mass-building exercise, using more weight can really help you build those stabilizer muscles that are so important for more basic movements.

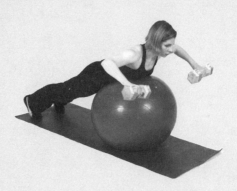

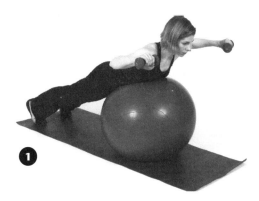

1

1 Rotate your lower arms up in front of you until they are parallel to the ground.

2 Lower the weights until your lower arms are about an inch short of hanging. Repeat the next rep without allowing your arms to rest.

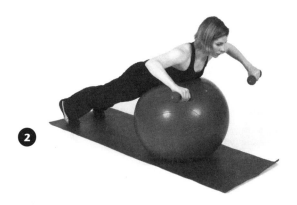

2

INTERMEDIATE

Perform this exercise very slowly. Take 10–15 seconds to perform each rep. Stop if you feel any impingement or pain.

preacher curls

This exercise is designed to allow you to isolate and train your biceps, particularly hitting the upper portion near your shoulders.

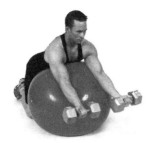

STARTING POSITION: Stand in front of the ball (or into the ball, depending on your size) and press your chest against it. You'll be resting on your knees with your feet shoulder width apart. You can bend at the waist, but maintain your spine in its neutral position throughout. Hold the weights with your palms facing away from you and the backsides of your upper arms against the ball. Your upper arms should be at an angle in relation to the ground. Avoid allowing the weights to contact the ground at any point during the rep (shorten your range of motion if necessary).

1 Using the power of your biceps, curl both weights up at the same time while pressing the backs of your arms against the ball, bringing them up until your palms are near your face and your lower arms are just short of perpendicular to the ground.

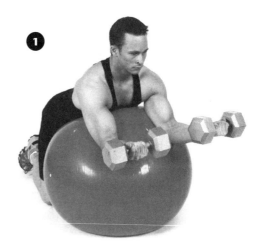

❶

variations

CONCENTRATION CURLS (BASIC)

Instead of working both arms simultaneously, try this version. Switch to the other arm after one set.

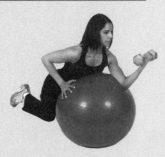

CONCENTRATION CURLS

Perform this variation while balanced on your toes, holding your body essentially in one line from your feet to the top of your head.

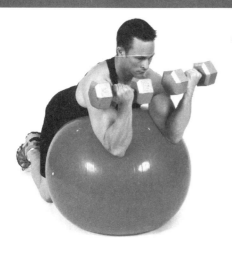

TIP

- If you have a barbell or E-Z-curl bar available, you may substitute it for dumbbells.
- To really work the top portion of the biceps, allow your upper arms to hang perpendicular to the ground throughout the entire set (you may need to use a large ball for this). If this is possible, you can do this as two separate exercises—one with upper arms perpendicular to the ground, the other with arms at about a 45-degree angle to the ground.

2 Squeeze your biceps at the top of the rep and hold for a beat.

3 Maintaining that contraction, lower the weights until your arms are almost fully extended.

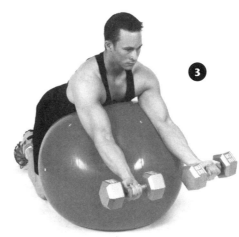

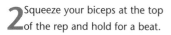

(INTERMEDIATE)

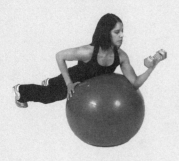

INTERMEDIATE/ADVANCED

Raise one leg behind you as you perform the set. Switch legs midway through the set. Perform one or two arms at a time.

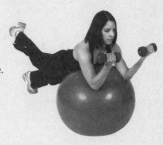

wrist curls (palm up)

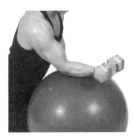

Often, the forearms are given little stimulation on their own and thus become the weak link in other movements. Working them directly can help overcome this, and performing this exercise one arm at a time really allows you to focus and concentrate on each arm.

STARTING POSITION: Kneel in front of (or into) your ball. Grasp a dumbbell in one hand and press the back of your forearm against the ball with your hand extending over the ball. Your lower arm should be close to parallel to the ground and relatively straight, but you can allow a 10- to 20-degree break at your elbow.

1 Bend your hand back and down toward the ground. Stop just short of the extent of your range of motion because taking the weight as deep as you can may lead to injury.

2 Pull the weight back up using the power of your forearm instead of your wrist joint. Concentrate on the feeling along your lower arm. Squeeze the weight at the top of the movement. Holding that tautness in your forearm, begin the next rep.

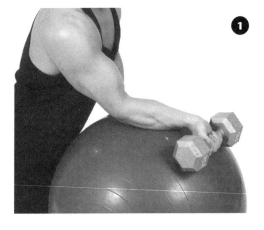

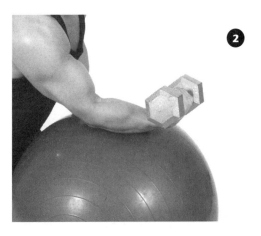

TIP

• Use a light weight, especially when you're new to this exercise, to allow your body to accommodate to it.

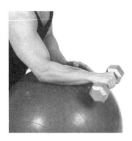

Very similar to the palms-up variety, this works your forearm from the opposite angle.

STARTING POSITION: Kneel in front of (or into) your ball. Grasp a dumbbell in your hand and place the inside of your forearm against the ball with your hand extending over the ball. Your arm should be relatively straight, but you can allow a 10- to 20-degree break at your elbow. Keep your forearm stationary throughout the movement.

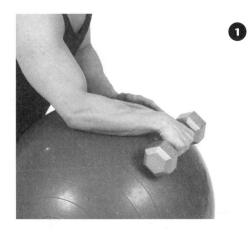

1

1 Bend your wrist down, taking it just slightly below parallel.

2 Roll your wrist up, bringing the weight up until your wrist is about 45 degrees above parallel to the ground (less if you have limited range of motion, more if you have excellent range of motion). Feel the stretch along your entire forearm. Holding your forearm taut, begin the next rep.

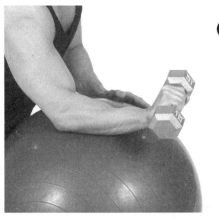

2

TIP

- Alternate sets of the palms-up and palms-down versions to create more balanced forearm strength.

planges

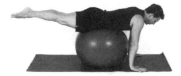

This is a great balance and stabilizing movement for developing shoulders.

STARTING POSITION: Place your midsection on the ball with your palms on the ground six to twelve inches in front of the ball. Keep your arms straight throughout the exercise. Raise your legs off the ground so that your body, from your feet to the top of your head, is in one plane approximately parallel to the ground. You may spread your legs apart or hold them close together, whichever feels more natural, as long as you keep them in that plane.

1 Without adjusting your hand position on the ground, roll forward on the ball, keeping the rest of your body in its plane. The ball will travel under you from your mid-abdomen down to your hip area.

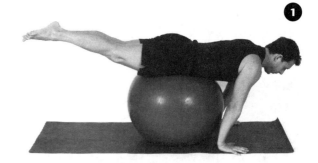

❶

variations

INTERMEDIATE

To intensify the work, hold the contraction longer rather than performing more reps.

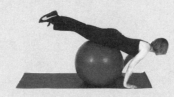

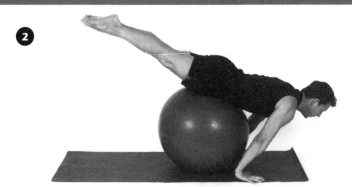

2

TIP

• The benefits of this exercise comes from holding the extended position rather than from performing reps. Start with just a couple of reps, and work up to only five or so.

2 Stop when your straight arms make about a 60-degree angle with the ground. Don't go too far or you'll lose your balance. You don't want to pitch forward and nose dive into the ground! Stabilize your body using the control of your shoulders. Squeeze them as you reach the end of your range of motion, holding for about five seconds.

3 By pressing out of your shoulders, roll back to your starting position with your arms perpendicular to the ground. Rest for a moment, if need be, and repeat.

3

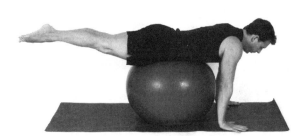

ADVANCED

Lighten the pressure of your hips against the ball. At the extended position, still keeping your body in one plane from your head to your hips, slowly elevate the lower body portion of that plane (so that the plane is no longer parallel to the ground). Your hips will get less support from the ball, and the demand on your shoulders will intensify.

dumbbell rows

This is one of the best lats developers that you can perform while using a balance ball.

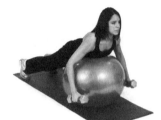

STARTING POSITION: From standing, place your lower chest on the ball so that you are facing downward with your feet shoulder width behind you. Balance on your toes, forming a slight incline from feet to head. Hold a dumbbell in each hand and extend your arms over the ball. Your palms can face each other, or you can rotate them out somewhat, whichever is more comfortable for you. Your spine should be aligned in its neutral position, with your hips just slightly lower than your shoulders. Take a wide stance and bend your knees so that you feel well stabilized.

1

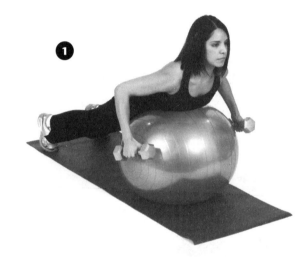

1 Bending at the elbow, pull the weights in a straight line up toward your armpits. Your elbows can travel slightly behind your back to allow you to get a good contraction at the top of the movement.

BASIC/INTERMEDIATE

Use heavier weights. The back is a strong muscle group and responds well to heavier weights. If you use the same weights for this one as you do for most of the other exercises described in this book, then your back, due to its relative potential strength, will be undertrained by comparison.

variations

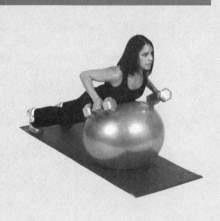

2

TIP

- It's easy to allow your shoulders to drop forward as you perform this exercise, but that over-stretches your traps and smaller back muscle—your goal is to stimulate your lats.

- Lower the weight with a three count, while you raise the weight with a one count and hold for one count. This meter is ideal for stimulating your target muscle while working against gravity.

3

2 Stop with the weights at chest level and hold that contraction for a second.

3 Keeping your shoulders rotated back, slowly lower the weights until your arms are fully extended (or as much as you can without contacting the ground or the ball). Repeat without pausing.

INTERMEDIATE

Make your upper body more parallel to the ground by raising your hips, bending at the waist but bending less at the knees. This hits your lats from a slightly different angle. Avoid allowing your head to bend down, out of neutral spinal position.

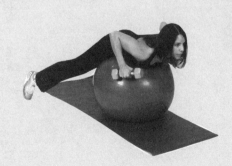

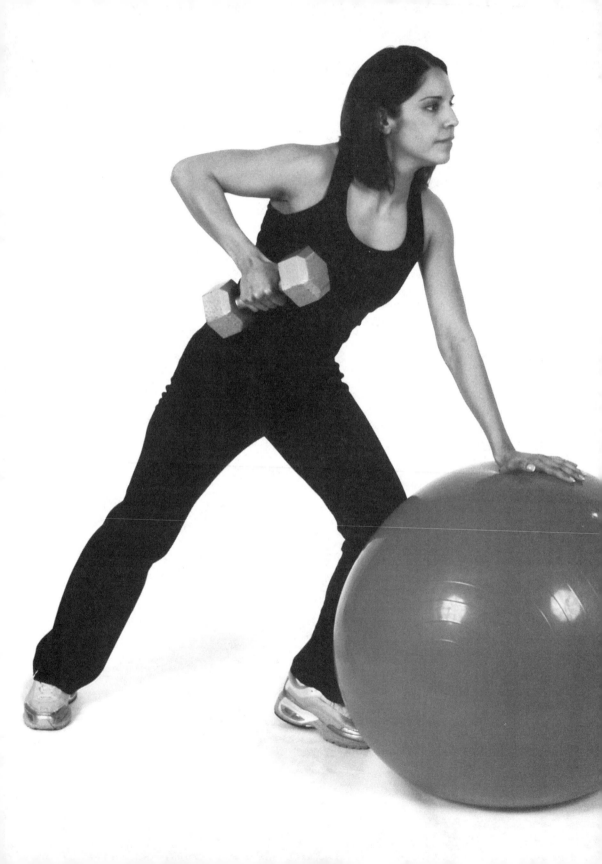

give yourself a hand: hands on the ball

When you perform exercises with your hand or hands on the ball, they become more difficult from a stabilizing standpoint as the ball supports more of your body weight. In some variations, you are only placing a small amount of weight against the ball to counterbalance the weight-training movement. In others, you are placing considerable weight against the ball, forcing your body to work hard to stabilize at the same time that you are performing a weight-lifting exercise. The exercises in this section target your chest, triceps, back or the entire body.

push-ups

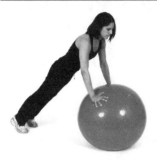

This is a terrific chest toner that requires more stabilizing, as well as a bit more strength, than the floor version.

STARTING POSITION: From standing, place your hands on the ball. Without moving your feet, roll the ball forward until your entire body is in plank position; hold onto the sides of the ball for balance. You will form a straight line from your feet to the top of your head as you balance on your toes. Place your hands as wide apart as the ball allows.

1 Lower your upper body to the ball by bending your elbows out to the side, still keeping your body from your feet to the top of your head in one plane. Feel the stretch in your chest as you lower yourself. Pause at the bottom of the movement.

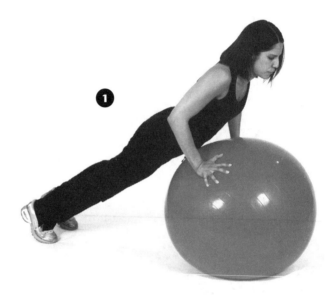

variations

BASIC	INTERMEDIATE/ADVANCED
If you're not ready to balance from your toes, try this exercise from your knees. Your body should form a straight line from your knees to the top of your head.	Perform push-ups with your feet on a bench, hands on the ball and your body parallel to the ground.

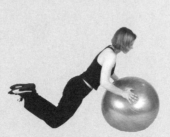

• Your back should be flat at the top of the movement, with your shoulders naturally retracted. Often, people will round their backs from side to side and push their shoulders forward. While this may make you feel more stable, it reduces the involvement of your pectorals, and thus the effectiveness of the movement.

2 Pressing through the heels, pads and fingers of your hands, push your body back up to the start position.

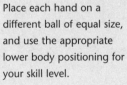

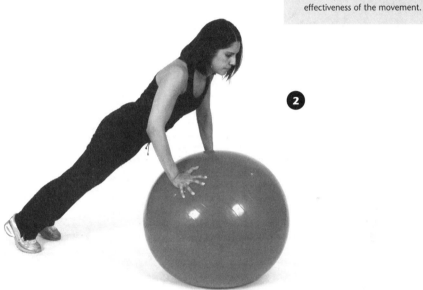

ADVANCED

Place each hand on a different ball of equal size, and use the appropriate lower body positioning for your skill level.

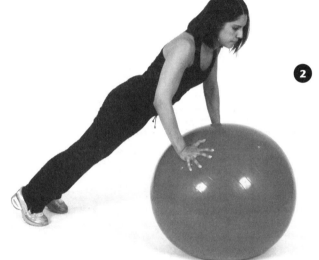

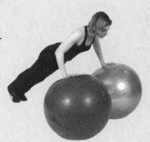

triceps kickbacks

This exercise allows you to stabilize your body with one hand while targeting the triceps on the opposite side.

STARTING POSITION: Stand facing the ball with your feet shoulder width apart. Bending at the waist, place one hand on the ball and rest a significant amount of your body weight against the ball. Your back can be parallel to the ground or angled, depending on your size and relationship to the ball you're using, but it should be In its neutral position throughout the movement. Hold a dumbbell in the hand not in contact with the ball and extend your working arm behind you so that your upper arm is parallel to the ground. Allow this arm to bend at the elbow so that the weight is hanging straight down or raised toward your shoulder.

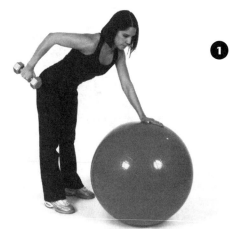

1 Holding the rest of your body stationary, extend the dumbbell behind you, moving only your lower arm (but using the power of your triceps along your upper arm). At the top of the movement, your entire arm should be close to parallel to the ground.

1

BASIC

You can help your stabilization by placing your knee (on the side of your body that is not holding the dumb-bell) against the ball.

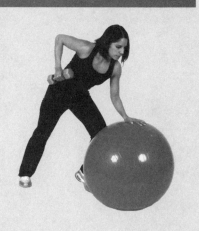

variations

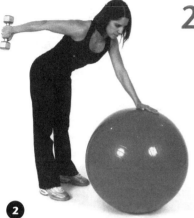

2 Squeeze your triceps and hold that contraction for a moment.

TIP

• Watch your balance as you extend your other arm behind you as you don't want to slide off the ball.

• For a little deeper contraction in your triceps, you can twist your wrist out and away from your body a bit. Do this as you reach the top of the movement.

3 Keeping your upper arm stationary, lower the weight, feeling the stretch along the backside of your upper arm. Bring your lower arm back down to just short of perpendicular. Stop at this point and go directly into the next rep. Perform all reps on one side, then switch to the other arm.

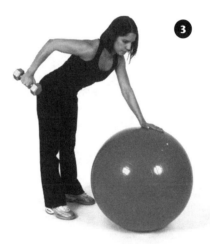

ADVANCED

While raising the weight behind you on one side, try raising the leg on the opposite side of your body. Try not to press too much of your weight against the ball, relying on this hand only for enough support to help you maintain your balance.

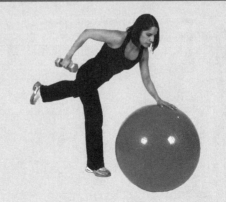

dumbbell rows

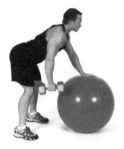

This movement targets the lats, the largest muscle of the back, as well as smaller back muscles. While this move is similar to the two-arm rowing motion, the one-arm version allows you a little more mechanical advantage so that you can use more weight.

STARTING POSITION: Stand facing the ball, feet shoulder width apart. Bending from the waist and slightly from the knees, place one hand on the ball. Your back should be flat, in its neutral position, with your head naturally extended, not bent up nor dropped down by your chest. Depending on the size of the ball, your back should be nearly parallel to the ground. Pick up a weight, allowing your arm to hang straight down perpendicular to the ground.

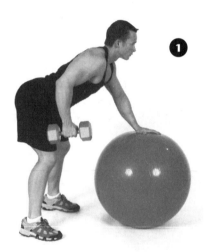

1 With your lower arm still hanging perpendicular to the ground, pull the weight up, allowing your elbow to travel slightly behind you. Try to keep your elbows from flaring out, and keep your back flat as you bring the weight up.

BASIC

You can try this with the same-side knee and hand on the ball for more stabilization.

variations

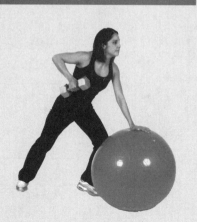

2

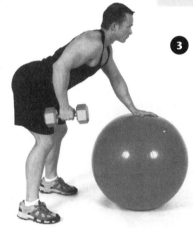

2 At the top, squeeze your lats (back muscles) for a moment.

3 Slowly lower your arm, making sure your shoulder doesn't drop. Feel the stretch as you work against gravity. Perform the reps for one side of your body, then switch and do the other.

3

ADVANCED

With only one hand on the ball, extend your same-side leg behind you. Using a much lighter weight, perform the exercise as before. This version is much more of a balance/stabilization movement than a muscle builder.

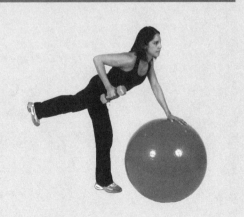

walk-arounds

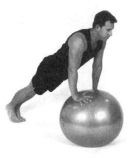

This is a great full-body movement that can be used as a warm-up or cool-down exercise, or you can integrate it into any of the other programs in this book. All versions of this move can be challenging.

STARTING POSITION: Place your feet close together as though you are going to do push-ups with your hands on the ball. Hold your body in plank position throughout the exercise; avoid letting your hips drop or raise up. Straighten your arms as much as possible.

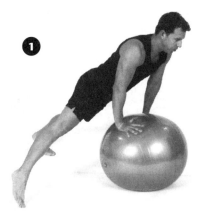

1

1 Take a wide step (about a yard) sideways with one foot. Maintain your balance on the ball.

variations

BASIC

This is a challenging movement, and just holding your body in this position without movement is an exercise. Try to work up to holding the position for 30–60 seconds.

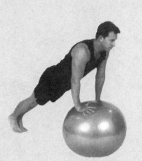

INTERMEDIATE

You may also bend your elbows so that your body is closer to the ball.

2

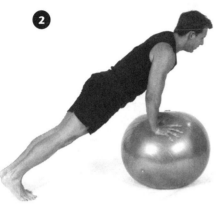

TIP

- Make certain to go both directions (clockwise and counterclockwise). Just doing one direction may leave you feeling like you've fully worked your body, but you should try both directions to work both sides of your body equally.

2 Move your second foot over so that your feet are again close together. Allow the ball to move underneath you and reposition your hands as necessary to maintain your balance and body control.

3 Continue to move in a circular direction around the ball (as opposed to moving left to right or vice versa).

3

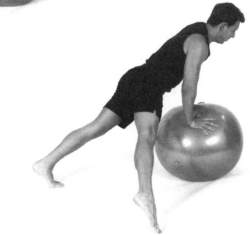

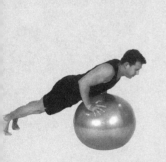

ADVANCED

Instead of placing your arms directly under your chest, extend them out just a bit so that they are angled into the ball, requiring your feet to be a little farther away from the ball. This will increase the work load on your upper body because of the increased distance from the ball.

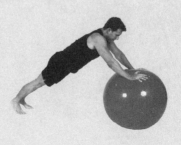

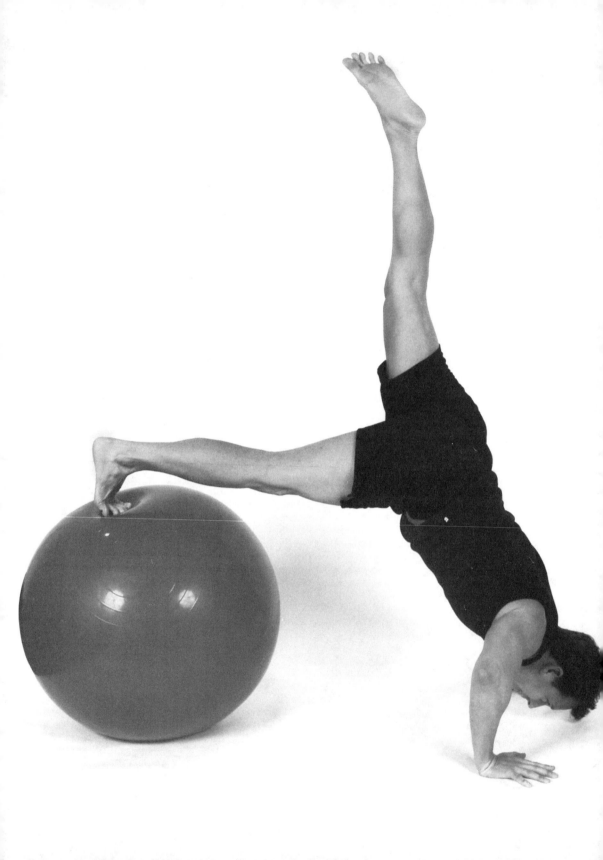

amazing feet
of strength:
feet on the ball

The unifying factor of the exercises in this section is
that they require you to place your feet on the ball,
but you primarily work your upper body. The
specific exercises target your chest, shoulders,
triceps or entire body. Often, these moves
require a great deal of strength. If placing
your feet on the ball for any of these moves
proves too challenging, you can modify
them by placing your lower legs, upper legs,
or even hips on the ball, whichever modifica-
tion best suits your strength, balance and
stabilization abilities.

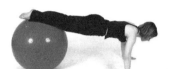

The strength demands of this version are greater than the stabilizing demands, making it an excellent toner and muscle-builder for the chest.

STARTING POSITION: Place your feet on the ball about shoulder width apart, with the tops of your feet being the primary contact with the ball. Place your hands on the floor slightly wider than your shoulders. Hold your body, from your ankles to the top of your head, in one plane. Resist sticking your butt up or allowing your hips to sag at any point during the set.

1 Slowly lower your body weight, keeping your body in one plane. Use the power of your pecs instead of emphasizing your triceps or shoulders. When you do this properly, not allowing gravity to bring your body down, you'll feel more of a stretch along your chest. Stop just short of letting any body part (your chest, your nose, your chin) touch the ground.

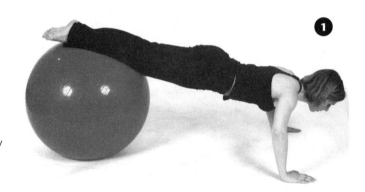

variations

BASIC/INTERMEDIATE

Place your feet farther apart on top of the ball. This shifts the angle at which you work your chest.

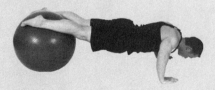

INTERMEDIATE

Place your hands slightly closer together so that they are slightly narrower than shoulder width. This will shift much of the weight from your chest to your triceps.

TIP

- If you are not strong enough for this position, you can place your upper legs against the ball. You'll work through a greater angle of motion, but the strength demands will be far less.

2

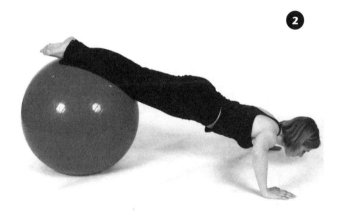

2 Using the muscular power of your chest, press back up until your arms are straight. At the top of the movement, your back should be flat, and your shoulders retracted (so that you are not hyperextended from the shoulder joint). Avoid locking out your arms and resting. Begin the next rep.

INTERMEDIATE/ADVANCED

Move the balance point from the tops of your feet to your toes.

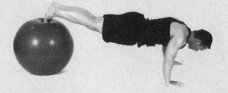

pike presses

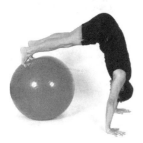

This is a challenging move that really works the shoulders as well as the traps and back. It imitates the feeling of an overhead press, only in reverse.

STARTING POSITION: Place your feet on the ball, and place your hands on the ground a few inches wider than your shoulders. Bend your body at the waist, holding your legs straight. Keep the ball as stable as possible. Your upper body should be relatively straight and almost perpendicular to the ground, making a 90-degree angle with your lower body (but you can cheat out a bit to reduce the strength and flexibility demands). Arms should be fully extended in the starting position.

1 Lower your body, bending at the elbows. Both arms should be essentially in one plane with your elbows flared out. Ideally, lower yourself until the top of your head nearly touches the ground (don't hit your head!), but you can go through a smaller range of motion if this is a challenging strength move for you.

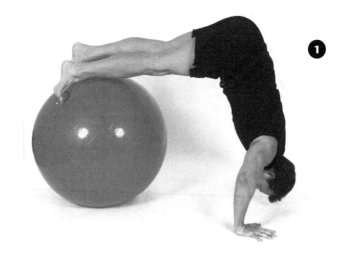

1

variations

BASIC

To make this exercise less strenuous, place your hands farther apart. In this position you'll work your middle delts a little more.

INTERMEDIATE

For more of a challenge, place your hands closer together, about shoulder width apart. These presses really target the front delts since your elbows stay closer to your body. You don't need to keep your elbows flared out in this position.

TIP

• Work to keep your body from lurching as you press up—keep it traveling smoothly in one plane. This will prevent you from over-recruiting support and/or back muscles, and keep the work focused on your target muscles.

2

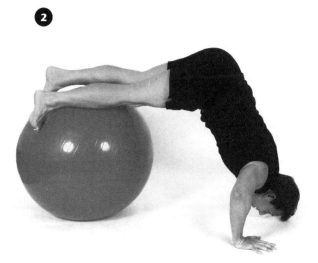

2 Press back up using the strength of your shoulders. Extend up until your arms are straight, but avoid locking them out at the top.

ADVANCED

Place only one foot on the ball, increasing the stabilizing demands of the movement.

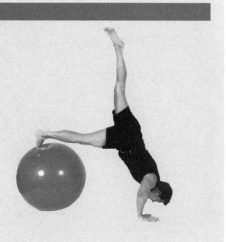

walk-arounds

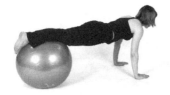

This is a great full-body movement, using the power of your upper body and the stabilization from your core as you travel all the way around the ball.

STARTING POSITION: Find a wide open space to perform this movement, with the ball in the center of that space. Place your feet or lower legs on the ball. Your hands should be comfortably shoulder width apart, and your body should form one line from your heels to the top of your head. Avoid allowing your hips to sag or your butt to stick up throughout the movement.

1 Move one hand out to the side, away from your body. Allow your elbow to bend a little with each arm movement.

2 Shift your body weight toward that hand and move your trailing arm into position so that your arms are once again about starting distance apart. Adjust your feet on the ball as necessary to maintain stability and positioning.

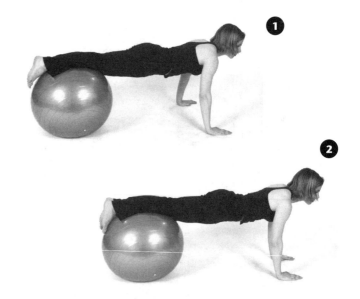

variations

BASIC

You can practice this move on the floor to begin with. The strength demands are still great, but you don't have to worry about stabilizing nearly as much.

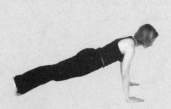

BASIC

Once you've gotten the hang of the movement from the floor, you may start with your upper legs, instead of your lower legs, on the ball as a way of working up to the full movement.

3 Continue to travel around the ball until you've traced a complete circle around the ball.

4 Reverse direction and make a complete circle the other way.

TIP

- Avoid overextending your shoulder joints (this will overwork small back muscles and your trapezius). Instead, hold your back flat throughout.
- Complete partial circles if you initially don't have the strength to perform full rotations. Work in both directions.

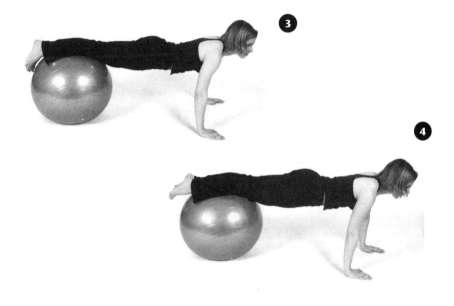

ADVANCED

Place your toes on the ball. This increases the stability work.

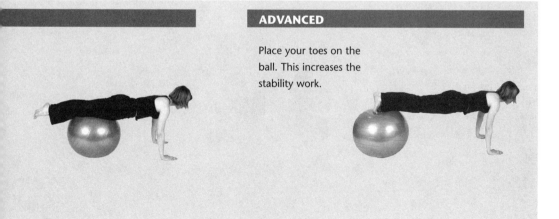

triceps dips

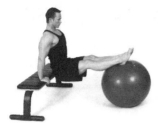

This is an excellent mass builder or toner for your triceps.

STARTING POSITION: Place your heels on the ball with your legs straight, and place your hands behind you on a bench or other stable piece of equipment or furniture. Your hands should be just far enough behind you that you can lower your butt below the level of the bench. Your hands should be spaced comfortably, about shoulder width apart.

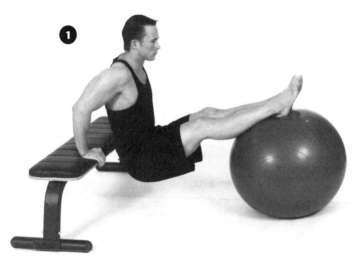

1 Lower your body weight using the power of your triceps. Do not let your elbows flare in or out; they should point directly behind you. Go as low as is comfortable, or stop at the point where your upper arms are parallel to the ground.

variations

BASIC

To decrease the range of motion and the amount of weight you lift, you can place your upper legs on the ball while placing your hands on the ground or on an object close to the ground (such as flat-ended weights or yoga blocks).

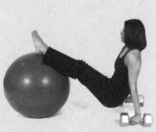

INTERMEDIATE

Place a dumbbell or two on your lap to increase the amount of weight your body must press.

TIP

• Try to avoid rounding your back, holding your shoulders slightly retracted.

2 Hold this position and feel a good stretch along the tops of your arms in the triceps. Activating from the triceps, press back up until your arms are fully extended but short of locking out. Squeeze your triceps at the top of the movement, and envision creating detail in the horseshoe portion of your triceps.

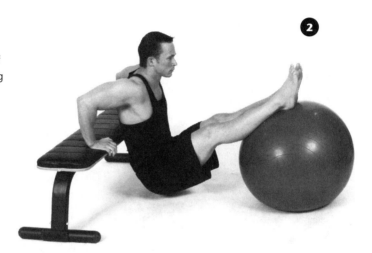

ADVANCED

Place your feet on the bench and your hands on the ball. Your legs can be bent for stability. As you dip down, your hips should drop lower than your feet. Ball positioning for this move can be tricky, so make certain that you are well stabilized.

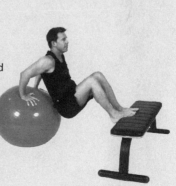

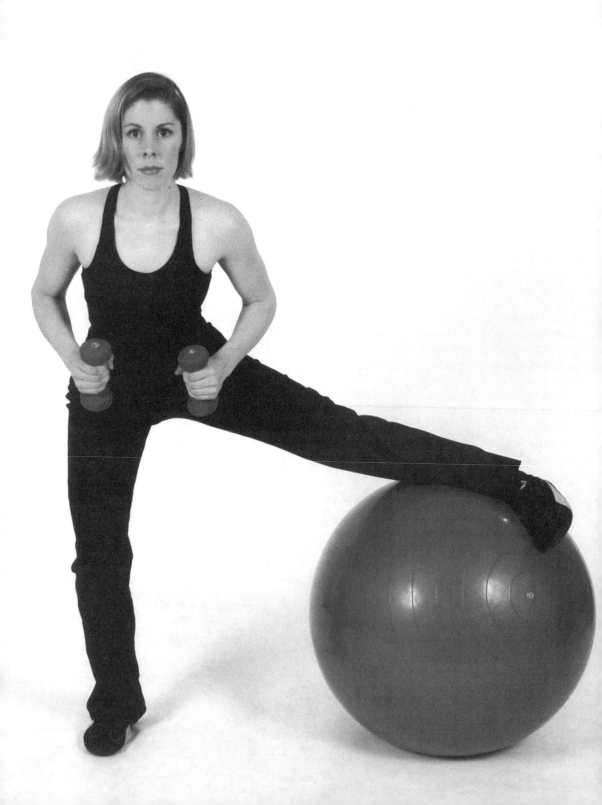

get a leg up:
leg strengtheners

The previous sections have mostly addressed upper-body movements. This section includes all the exercises that most directly target your lower body. As such, the starting position relative to the ball varies considerably from one exercise to another. For some movements, you are lying on the ball, for others you place the ball between yourself and the wall, for still others you hold the ball or use it for stability. Again, it only goes to show just how versatile this weights-and-ball workout can be!

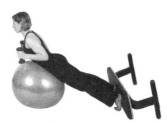

This exercise works your spinal erectors, glutes and hamstrings and helps build a strong core. It's a great exercise to balance abdominal training, and it's good for those who have back problems.

STARTING POSITION: Place your hips or lower abdominals on the ball, near a wall. Press your heels against the wall, with the balls of your feet on the ground, about shoulder width apart. Your body should form one long line from your feet to the top of your head. Grasp a dumbbell in each hand at your upper chest.

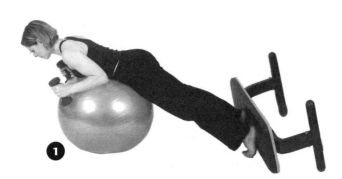

1 Keeping your spine in its neutral position, slowly bend from the waist, keeping your legs straight. This can be challenging, so proceed carefully. Bend as low as is comfortable. If you're flexible, you may be able to bend down until your head is near the ground. The size of the ball you work with may also impact your range of motion. If you lack flexibility, you may not be able to get your upper body parallel to the ground (see the Tip if this is the case). At the bottom of the movement, you should feel a nice stretch along your hamstrings and glutes.

variations

BASIC

If holding the dumbbell makes this move too difficult, you can attempt it without holding any weight at all.

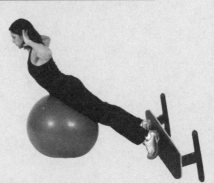

INTERMEDIATE

To intensify the stretch and shift it a bit, place your feet closer together. This requires even more flexibility and stability.

2 Pulling from your hamstrings and glutes, raise your body back up until you are just short of your starting position. Contract your working muscles and then, holding them tight, go directly into the next rep.

TIP

- If keeping your legs straight is too challenging, you can widen your stance and bend your knees slightly. This will better allow you to maintain your neutral spinal position, which is crucial for targeting the proper muscles and avoiding injury.
- If the ball feels unstable underneath you, you can place your hands on the ball as you perform the movement.

2

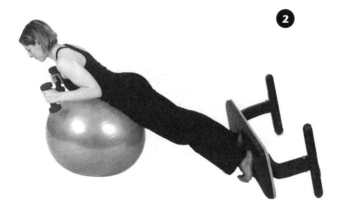

INTERMEDIATE/ADVANCED

To increase the difficulty, move away from the wall so that you must stabilize without the wall's support.

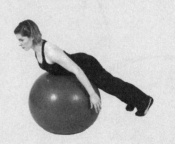

reverse back extensions

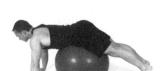

Similar to back extensions, the reverse version targets the spinal erectors a bit more. The spinal erectors are an important muscle to develop because they are often the weak-link muscle that leads to injury or lower back discomfort related to ordinary movement or exercise.

STARTING POSITION: With your hips or lower abdomen on the ball, bend at the waist in order to place your hands on the ground. For the best range of motion, your hips should be slightly higher than your shoulders—you can bend your arms to get this position. Keep your spine in its neutral position—your body should form one line from your butt to the top of your head. Your toes should just touch the ground at the start of the exercise.

1 Holding your legs straight, raise them off the ground. Bring them up until your lower body is parallel to the ground. You can raise them a little more for added range of motion and work, but avoid allowing your back to arch. At the top of the movement contract the muscles in the middle of your lower back and your glutes.

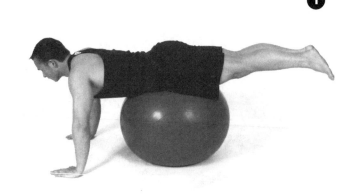

1

variations

INTERMEDIATE

Instead of balancing from your hands, try placing your forearms on the ground and performing the exercise from this position. You may extend your legs above parallel for a fuller range of motion.

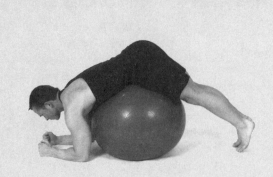

TIP

• Throughout this movement, imagine your spine holding its neutral position while you think about elongating your body as much as you can. Elongating your body will help improve your posture and keep your spine in its proper position at the same time.

2 Holding the muscles in the middle of your lower back tight, slowly begin to lower your legs—avoid allowing gravity to pull your legs back down to the ground. Stop just before your toes touch the ground and go into your next rep.

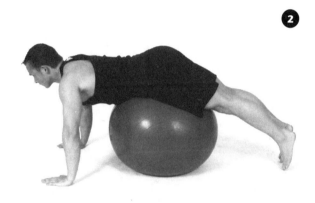

2

ADVANCED

Once you have experience with this movement, try grasping a small dumbbell between your feet (you may want to wear shoes to protect your feet). Raise your legs carefully, making certain not to drop the weight on the ground (or worse!) on yourself if you raise your legs above parallel.

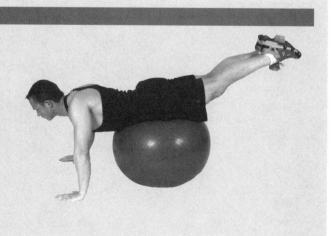

hamstrings curls

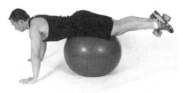

Hamstrings are the muscles at the backs of the legs. Often, these muscles are underutilized in other legs workouts, so including an exercise to target them directly is a great idea for balanced development.

STARTING POSITION: Place your hips and upper legs on the ball and put your hands on the ground for stability. Your feet should be off the ground. Hold a weight between your feet and press your feet together, allowing the head of the dumbbell to rest on the soles of your shoes (this can be tricky—you may want a partner to help position the weight). At the starting point, your body should form one long line from the dumbbell at your feet to the top of your head.

1 Holding your body straight from your knees to the top of your head, curl your legs up until your lower legs are above your knees and just short of perpendicular to the ground. (Your lower legs are the only part of your body that should move during this exercise.) Think about pulling from the back center of your legs and contracting your hamstrings as you reach this peak position.

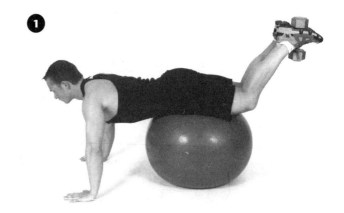

1

variations

BASIC

If you have difficulty balancing the weight, or simply to make the exercise a little easier, you can use ankle weights instead of a dumbbell.

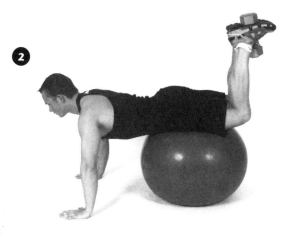

2 Hold that contraction for a moment. At the top, make certain that you bend your ankles slightly so that the dumbbell continues to rest on the soles of your shoes. Pay attention to your feet and the dumbbell to avoid dropping the weight on the floor—or worse, on yourself.

3 Slowly lower the weight, feeling the stretch in your hamstrings, and move into the next rep.

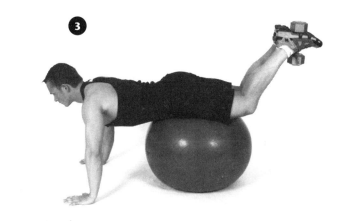

TIP

- Avoid arching your back or changing your upper-body positioning throughout the exercise.
- Avoid taking the weight past perpendicular toward your butt.

INTERMEDIATE

This exercise is plenty challenging as it is, but if you want to increase the challenge somewhat, use a slightly heavier weight than you do for most exercises. Because of the risk of dropping the weight, make certain to maintain control throughout the entire set.

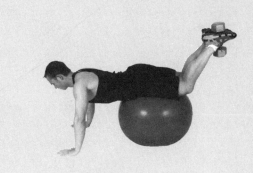

stiff-legged deadlifts

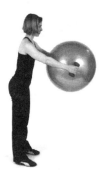

These are great for developing the hamstrings, glutes and spinal erectors.

STARTING POSITION: Stand upright. Holding a weight in each hand, palms facing inward, squeeze the ball between your forearms or the heels of your palms. Extend your arms out nearly parallel to the ground so that the ball doesn't contact your body. You can bend your knees just a little bit—about a five-degree bend to help protect your lower back. If you are flexible and have a strong lower back, you can perform the exercise with straight legs.

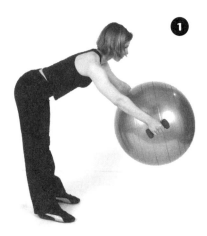

1 Bending forward only from the waist, lower the top half of your body, keeping your spine in its neutral position throughout. Allow your hands and the ball to travel out in front of you so that the ball doesn't touch your body. Stop just before the ball touches the ground—if you're flexible, you may need to hold the ball nearly from the bottom. At this point, the upper part of your body should be close to parallel to the ground.

variations

BASIC

To lessen the intensity, try this exercise with only the ball until you are strong enough to use both the ball and weights. (You can also bend your arms at the elbows.)

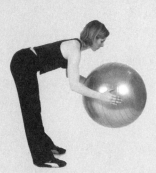

INTERMEDIATE/ADVANCED

Try this with one leg at a time—it's very challenging. Hold the ball and, keeping your torso as square as possible, bend forward on one leg.

2

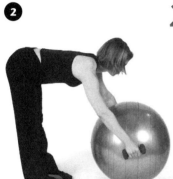

2 Feel the stretch along the hamstrings and glutes.

3

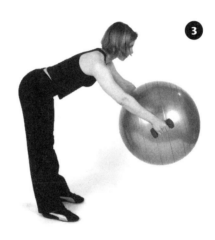

3 Pulling with the hamstrings and glutes, begin to raise your upper body back to the start position. Stop just short of vertical and go into the next rep.

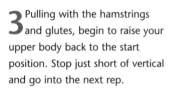

ADVANCED

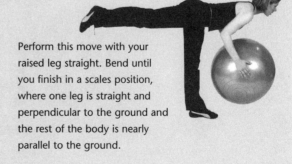

Perform this move with your raised leg straight. Bend until you finish in a scales position, where one leg is straight and perpendicular to the ground and the rest of the body is nearly parallel to the ground.

wall squats

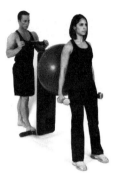

This is a great exercise for working your legs while improving your posture and balance at the same time. Squats are the best overall legs developer, and this ball-and-wall version also emphasizes stability, really allowing you to target your quads.

STARTING POSITION: Place the ball between your lower back and a wall. Stand with your feet about shoulder width apart, just slightly out in front of your body, and grasp a dumbbell in each hand. Your arms should hang down by your sides.

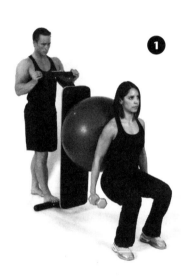

1

1 Squat down, allowing the balance ball to roll against your back. Keeping your shoulders rolled back and your spine in its neutral position, allow the weights to travel down toward the ground. Feel the stretch in your glutes and across your quads. Lower your hips until your upper legs are parallel to the ground.

variations

WALL SQUAT CURLS

You can perform a curl as you squat down. This is an efficient combination move that targets both the legs and upper body. It is included in many of the workouts.

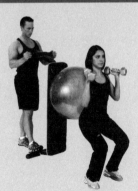

INTERMEDIATE/ADVANCED

Perform this exercise one leg at a time. This is significantly more challenging, and you should first attempt it without dumbbells. Use your arms for balance, if needed. At first, stop before you reach parallel as you are teaching your body to accommodate to this movement. Repeat on the other side.

2 Press through both your heels and the balls of your feet and begin to roll back up slowly, with control. Stop short of locking out your knees, and begin your next rep

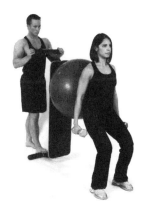

2

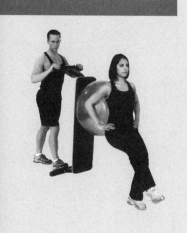

ADVANCED

Perform one-legged squats while holding a dumbbell in each hand at your shoulders.

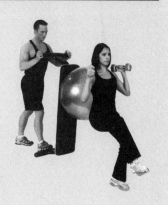

lunges

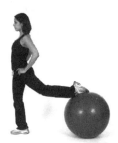

Lunges are not only a great legs developer, but they help give your legs an elongated appearance as they add tone and definition. The unilateral (one leg at a time) element of the movement helps you develop balance and control. It's an excellent movement for enhancing everyday functionality.

STARTING POSITION: Stand with the ball behind you on the floor, and extend one leg back and place the top of your foot on the ball. Your upper body should be upright, with your spine in its neutral position and your shoulders rotated back; maintain this form throughout the exercise.

1 Slowly lower your hips by bending your front knee. Allow your back leg to roll on the ball, if needed, and lower your hips toward the ground. Lower your body as much as you can (and as much as the ball allows) while still maintaining control and balance. Feel the stretch along the top of your back leg and along the backside of your front leg.

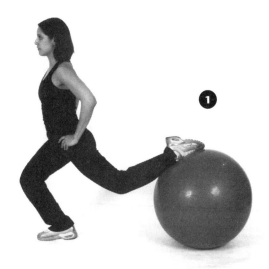

variations

INTERMEDIATE

Hold a weight in each hand to increase the strength demands on your legs.

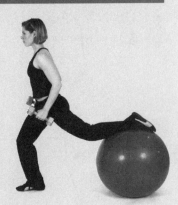

INTERMEDIATE/ADVANCED

Place only the toes of your back foot on the ball. This will deepen the demand on your leg muscles and require more stability and balance.

TIP

• Don't allow your upper body to lurch during the movement. This undercuts the effectiveness of the exercise and encourages injury to the lower back, as well as tending to throw you off balance.

2 Press back up through the foot that's on the floor, concentrating on using the power of your quads, calves, hamstrings and glutes.

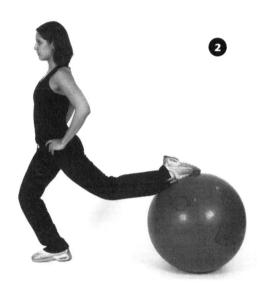

2

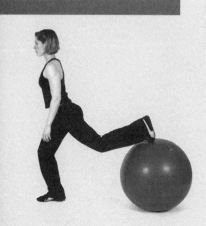

ADVANCED

Try the second challenge while holding weights.

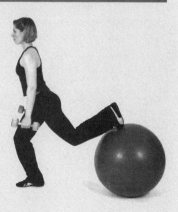

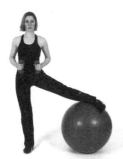

The muscles on the interior and exterior of your legs tend to get less muscular stimulation than the major muscles such as quads and hamstrings. Yet, the minor muscles are often the ones that are overtaxed when you place atypical demands on your lower body. Using the ball to perform this exercise encourages the strengthening of the muscles of the inner and outer thighs.

STARTING POSITION: Stand beside your ball and place the inside of your lower leg on top, or just on the far side, of the ball. Keep your spine in its neutral position throughout this movement. Hold a dumbbell in each hand.

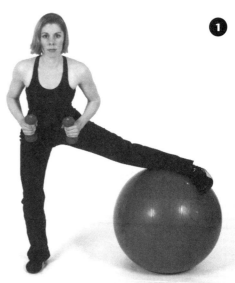

1

1 Bend the knee of the leg that's in contact with the ground and drop your hips toward the floor. Push your hips back just a bit and you can allow your whole torso, from your pelvis upward, to tilt forward a little— as long as you keep your spine in its neutral position. At first, you may not be able to lower your body very much, but eventually work up to the point where you are lowering your body so that the leg on the ball is nearly parallel to the ground.

INTERMEDIATE/ADVANCED

Stand even farther from the ball, allowing only your foot and ankle to contact the ball.

variations

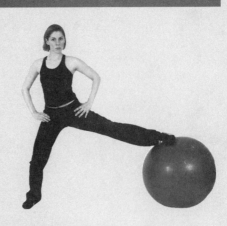

2 Press back up through the foot that's in contact with the floor, also concentrating on using the power of your leg muscles.

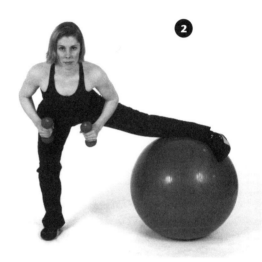

ADVANCED

Hold a dumbbell in front of your body, and allow it to travel down between your legs as you perform side lunges. (You can still allow your whole torso to tilt forward a bit, as long as your spine remains in its neutral position throughout.)

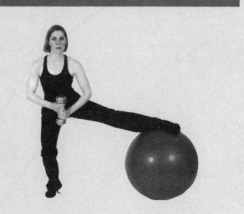

lateral leg raises

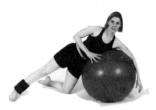

This move is excellent for providing toning for the upper legs, particularly inner and outer thighs. Incorporating variations in your workouts further enhances this benefit.

STARTING POSITION: From your knees, place one side against the ball, allowing your arm to wrap over the top of the ball to help control your body weight. Extend the opposite leg (with an ankle weight) so that the edge of your foot is just touching the ground.

1 Holding your opposite leg straight, raise it until it is parallel (or a little higher than parallel) to the ground.

1

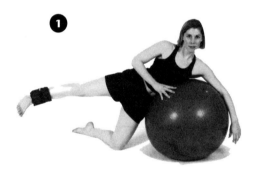

BASIC/INTERMEDIATE

Increase the intensity by slowing down the pace, increasing the weight (you can use two ankle weights on one leg) or extending the length of the hold at the top.

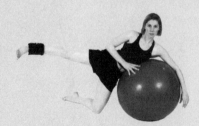

variations

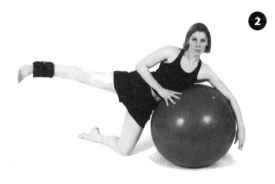

2 At the top of the movement, tense the muscles across the outside of your raised leg. Hold that position for a couple seconds.

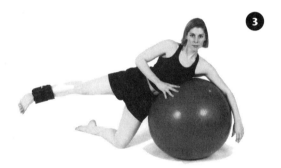

3 Begin to lower your leg, keeping the tension along the outside of that leg. Lower your leg, but stop short of allowing your foot to touch the ground. Complete all the reps for that side of your body, then do the same for the other side.

INTERMEDIATE

From the top position, bring your knee out in front of you, keeping your leg essentially parallel to the ground. This will incorporate a little more glutes work and increase the stability demands.

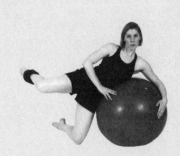

seated calf raises

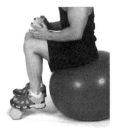

In some ways, calves are worked as much as any muscle in the body—you use them every time you take a step. But they are often underutilized in terms of their strength. The purpose of this exercise is to strengthen your calves using a greater range of motion and weight, as opposed to working them through many repetitions, as you do every day while walking.

STARTING POSITION: Sit on the ball with your feet on a stable object such as a yoga block, a block of wood or a stable weight. Rest a dumbbell on your legs near your knees. Use only your hands to keep them in place—do not use them to assist with moving the weights.

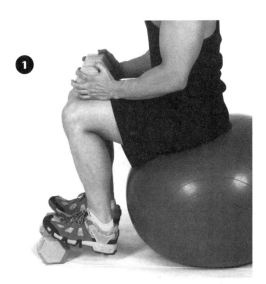

1 Moving only your ankle joint, slowly allow your heels to dip lower than the surface of the object on which your legs are positioned. Feel a good stretch along the backs of your lower legs.

variations

BASIC/INTERMEDIATE

Perform this movement one leg at a time, using one dumbbell.

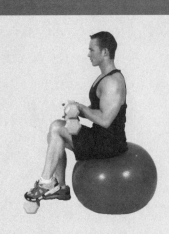

2

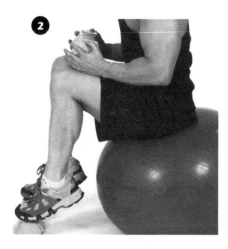

3

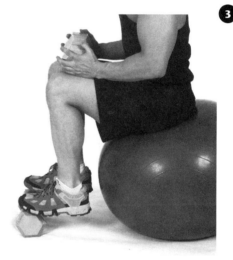

2 Pressing through the balls of your feet, raise your heels until they are an inch or two above the surface. Contract the muscles at the backs of your lower legs and hold for a couple of seconds.

3 Still holding the muscles tight, lower your ankles back to the starting position and perform the next rep.

ADVANCED

Place a dumbbell on your working leg and raise your other leg off the ground. This requires core stability as well as muscular strength.

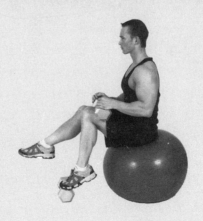

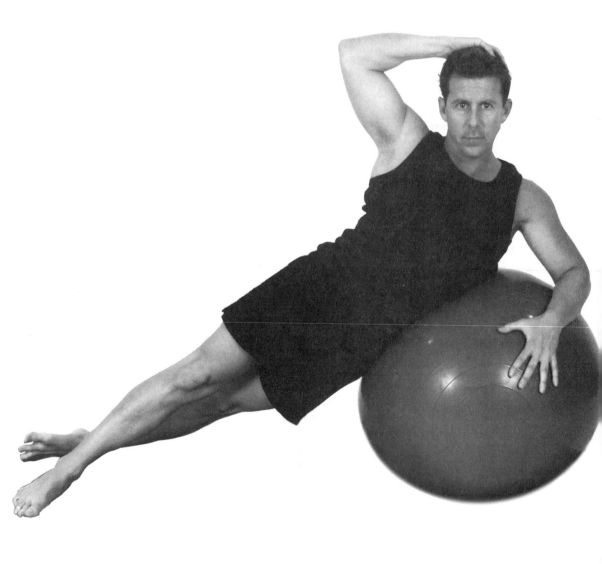

core concerns:
abs movements

One of the greatest benefits of the weights-on-the-ball workout is that most of the exercises require you to use your core strength for stability. While this indirectly targets abdominal development and enhances the overall appearance and strength of your midsection, it's also a good idea to directly target this part of your body as well. The following abdominal and core exercises do just that from a variety of angles and position—lying on the ball or the floor, seated on the ball or with your side against the ball. Integrating some or all of these exercises into your training will help you develop the midsection you've always wanted.

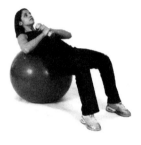

Crunches on the ball are not only the most basic balance-ball abs movement, but they're also more effective than the floor version because you can more directly target your abdominal muscles.

STARTING POSITION: Sit on the ball and slowly drop your hips as you move your feet forward. This will allow you to safely get into place on the ball. To begin the movement, the upper part of your butt and lower back should be in contact with the ball, and your feet should be firmly planted on the floor. Your shoulders should be slightly higher than your hips and your spine should be in its neutral position. Make certain that your body weight sinks into the ball enough that the ball doesn't shoot out behind you as you perform the exercise (even if you're home alone, this can prove embarrassing!). Hold a dumbbell up at your chest with both hands.

1 Holding your lower body stationary, curl your torso up, focusing on feeling a tightening in your abs. Curl until you feel a deep contraction within your abs (you don't have to come all the way up—sometimes a range of motion of only a few inches is enough to generate an effective contraction).

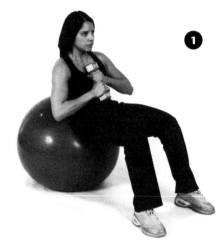

1

variations

BASIC

Instead of doing this exercise with a weight, place your hands behind your neck, or fold them across your chest.

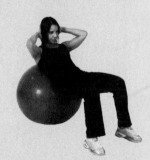

INTERMEDIATE

Perform crunches with a slight twist at the top of the movement. This will activate the obliques as well as your abs.

2 Maintaining that contraction, lower your body back to the start position, feeling the stretch in your abs.

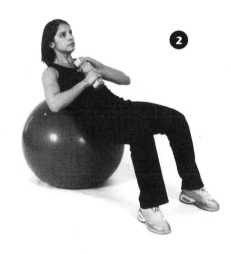

2

ADVANCED

Perform half a set with one foot off the ground, then switch feet and perform the second half of the set with the other foot off the ground.

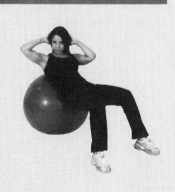

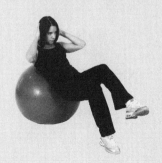

abs crunches (feet on the ball)

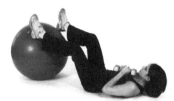

Abs crunches are one of the most basic movements for developing your midsection. This version allows you to stabilize your upper body more from the hips. Placing your feet on the ball further enhances stabilization work.

STARTING POSITION: Lie on the floor with your heels resting on top of the ball. Your lower legs should be parallel to the ground (widen your legs a bit if the ball is too large to allow for this in the center), and your upper legs should be nearly perpendicular to the ground, angling slightly toward the ball. Using both hands, hold a weight across your chest.

1 Pulling from the core of your body, not from your neck, begin to roll your upper torso toward your knees and the ball. As the muscles of your abdomen shorten, deepen the contraction by squeezing them down toward the floor. At the peak of the movement, your head and shoulders may only be a couple of inches off the floor. Hold that position for a couple seconds.

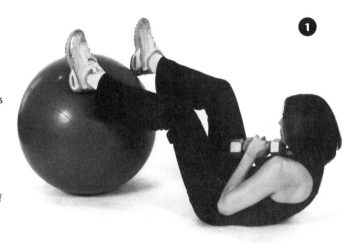

1

BASIC

Instead of holding a weight, fold your arms across your chest, or place your hands behind your neck with your elbows flared open.

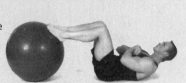

BASIC/INTERMEDIATE

For a little more challenge, try holding the weight behind your neck with both hands.

variations

2 Still holding your abdominals tight, begin to stretch back to the floor. At the bottom of the movement, do not release your abs. This allows you to rest and reduces the effectiveness of the exercise. Instead, stop just short of your starting position and go directly into your next rep.

TIP

• Focus more on the feeling in your abs than on the range of motion. When you correctly perform abdominal exercises, regardless of your physical conditioning, you should be working hard enough that you can't perform more than 15–20 reps. If you can do more reps than this, work harder and more slowly on individual reps.

• All of these moves can also incorporate a twist to activate your obliques.

2

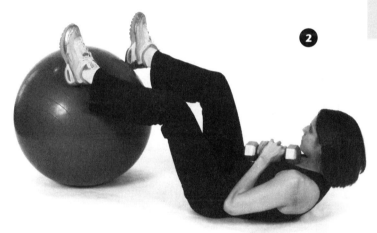

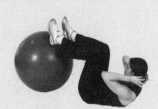

INTERMEDIATE

Place the ball against a wall and place your feet against the other side of the ball, pinning the ball between your feet and the wall. Now perform crunches. This variety requires a little more abdominal stability because you must engage your abs throughout to hold the ball in place.

roll-up crunches

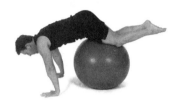

At first, this is a tricky movement. However, once you have mastered the stabilizing aspect of it, you will be able to very effectively target your abs.

STARTING POSITION: Lie face down on the ball. Place the tops of your upper thighs on the ball and support your body weight with your hands out in front of you on the ground. Hold your arms straight and slightly wider than shoulder width apart throughout the movement.

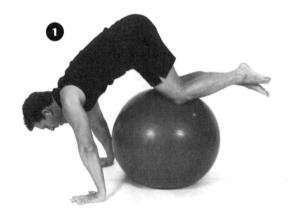

1 Without moving your hands, roll your knees toward your arms, allowing the ball to travel under you so that at the peak position it is under your lower legs at your knees. As you bring your knees in, your lower back and butt should curl upward.

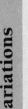
variations

INTERMEDIATE

As you bring your knees close to your hands, twist to the side a little to recruit your obliques (the muscles on your sides) a bit more. Be careful not to lose your balance on the ball. Perform all reps on one side, then the other; or, alternate one side then the other.

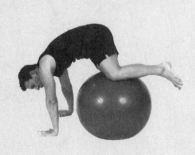

2

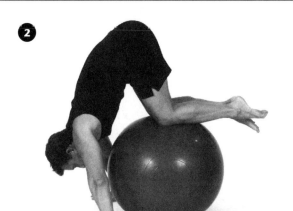

TIP

- Contracting your abs can be tricky—at first, your primary concern should be to maintain body control, balance and stability so that you don't slip off the ball. Later, as your skill improves, you can begin to target your abs more.

3

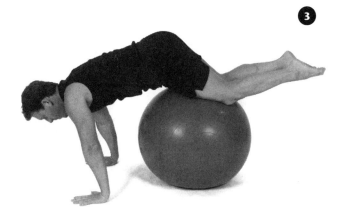

2 At the top of the movement, contract your abs and hold the contraction for a moment.

3 Slowly begin to roll the ball back, extending your legs behind you until you return to the plank starting position.

ADVANCED

Place your feet on the ball to create a longer range of motion, forcing your body to stabilize more. Perform the straight-on or twist variation.

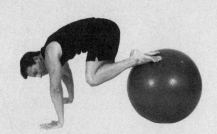

reverse crunches

While most crunches tend to better work the upper portion of the abdominals, reverse crunches tend to better work the lower portion. Often, this lower part of a person's abdominals is the most difficult part to develop. Incorporating exercises that directly target this part of the body is great for total core development.

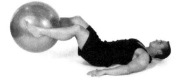

STARTING POSITION: Lie with your back on the floor and your balance ball positioned between your lower legs. Squeeze the ball with your legs and hold it just off the ground. Your knees should be slightly bent. Place your arms at your sides with your palms on the ground to help stabilize your body.

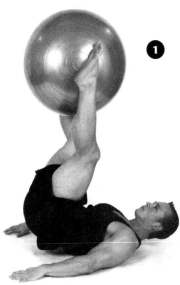

1 Curl your hips off the ground, bringing the ball up and toward your upper body. You can bend your knees more to help contract your abdominals. Hold that contraction for a moment.

variations

INTERMEDIATE

To increase the resistance, strap on ankle weights.

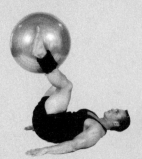

ADVANCED

Place your back on a second ball and stabilize your body by holding onto something stationary behind you.

TIP

• You can also place your arms overhead and hold onto a stationary item, such as a heavy piece of furniture. This opens up your abs, allowing you to take them through a greater range of motion, stretching them a bit more.

2 Slowly lower your hips and stretch your legs back out. Make certain to keep the ball from contacting the ground at the end of the movement since this will encourage you to rest, under-cutting the benefit of the exercise.

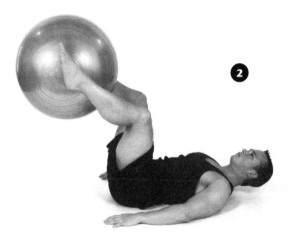

ADVANCED

Add ankle weights to increase the resistance. This is very challenging.

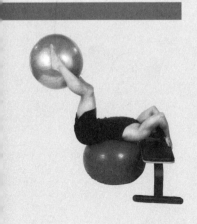

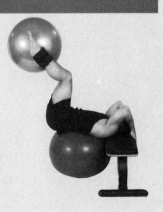

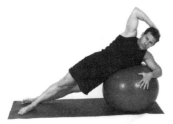

This is a great movement for developing your obliques—as well as helping to enhance your balance and stabilization.

STARTING POSITION: Lie with one side of your body pressed against the ball. Place the arm on the side of the body that contacts the ball on the ball. Place the other arm at the back of your head, with your elbow aiming upward towards the ceiling. With your legs straight, stabilize your body by moving one foot forward and the other back, allowing the downward edge of each foot to rest against the ground. For the most part, your body should be in one plane, splitting through the ball.

1 Roll your upper body up, stretching your head toward the ceiling as you also imagine your elbow curling toward your hip. The range of motion is quite small—you may only move your upper body a couple of inches from the starting point. As you reach the peak of the movement, crunch down on your side abdominals that are open to the ceiling (not the ones in contact with the ball). Squeeze these muscles for a moment.

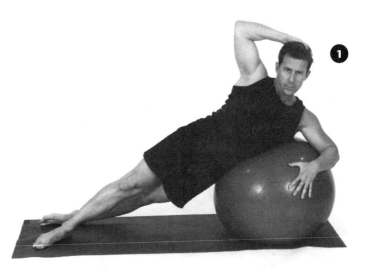

variations

INTERMEDIATE

Bring your legs together with your upper foot on top of the lower. This will force you to stabilize more and increase the balance demand on your body.

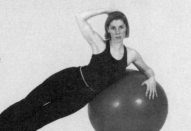

ADVANCED

Raise the top leg up off the lower stabilizing leg and hold it parallel to the ground.

2 Holding the side abdominals taut, stretch your body down until it is just short of your starting position. Perform reps on one side, then repeat on the other.

TIP

• At first, the balance elements of this movement are difficult and may prevent you from feeling much of contraction. As your balance improves—and as your overall abdominal strength improves from your program—your ability to effectively use this movement as an abdominal trainer will also improve.

2

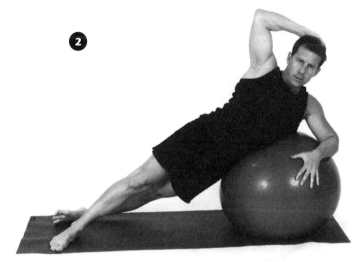

ADVANCED

Bring your upper knee in and curl your torso toward your knee—be careful to maintain balance so you don't flop off of the ball. This movement is slightly different from the other variations, targeting your six-pack abdominals a little more than the other two challenges.

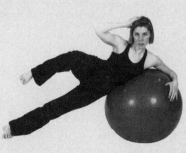

cross-body twists

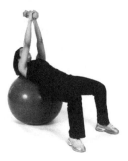

This is an excellent weight-and-ball movement for developing the upper muscles at your sides.

STARTING POSITION: Lie with your upper back against the ball. Place your feet shoulder width apart. You can allow your hips to dip just slightly below the plane formed between your knees and shoulders. Hold one dumbbell in both hands. Extend the dumbbell so that it is above your upper chest.

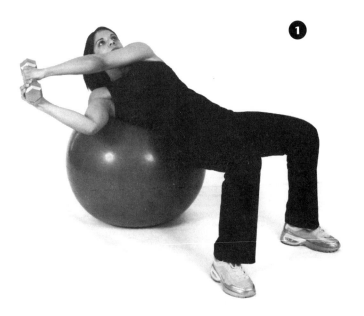

1

1 Slowly rotate your torso and move the weight out to one side. Maintain your spine in its neutral position and keep your neck extended with your gaze to the ceiling. Feel a good stretch at your sides, engaging both.

variations

BASIC/INTERMEDIATE

Slowly, and with control, rotate your upper torso with the weight, allowing your head to turn with your body. This variation will work the muscles of your sides through a greater range of motion.

2 Slowly rotate your torso and the weight back up through the starting position and over to the other side. Make certain to work within a range of motion that's comfortable for you.

TIP

• Avoid using momentum to move the weight. This exercise can provide a fairly dynamic stretch, especially at first. Keeping the weight light and moving it slowly will help you work your target muscles and avoid injury.

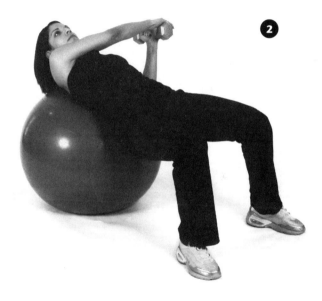

2

INTERMEDIATE

Extend your legs so that they are straight and close together, allowing only your heels to touch the ground.

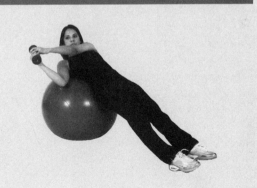

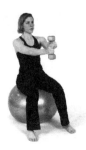

Though similar to the side twists with your back on the ball, the seated position targets your core a little differently.

STARTING POSITION: Sit on the ball with your feet shoulder width apart. Hold a weight with both hands out in front of you, with your arms at shoulder height—hold the weight perpendicular to the ground, grasping it by the upper head with both hands. Sit up as tall as possible, elongating your spine and neck, holding them in the neutral position.

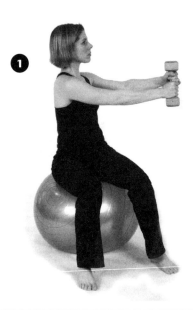

1 Stabilizing yourself from the core and with your feet solidly planted on the ground, twist to one side, keeping your arms extended and at shoulder height. Squeeze your abs, focusing on the abs on the side you've turned to. At the same time, feel the stretch on the opposite side.

variations

BASIC/INTERMEDIATE

Perform all reps for one side of your body, then perform all the reps for the other, stopping at the center point after each rep. This will place more demand on the working side since you allow it no rest time between reps.

INTERMEDIATE

Narrow your stance—the narrower stance will allow for greater range of motion and require more stabilization of your core.

TIP

• To make this exercise effective, you must really concentrate on intensifying the contraction in your abdominals. You'll get far better results this way than if you merely just take your body through the range of motion.

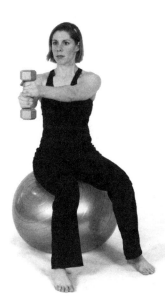

2 Rotate back through the center and over to the other side, crunching down on the other side of your abs.

ADVANCED

Perform the exercise with your feet off the ground.

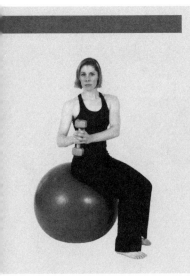

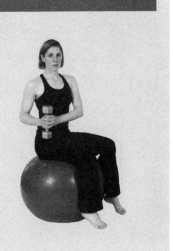

hip raises

This exercise targets the smaller muscles in your hips and inner thighs.

STARTING POSITION: Lie flat on the ground with your feet against the ball. Secure the ball against a wall so that it is pinned between the wall and your feet. Your upper legs should angle toward the ball and your lower legs can be parallel, or a little above or below, depending on the size of the ball. All in all, the ball should be a foot or so beyond your butt. Extend your arms to your sides, contacting the floor.

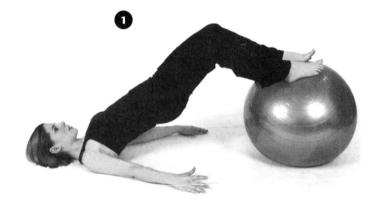

1 Slowly raise your hips up off the floor—take them up until your body is nearly straight from knees to shoulders. At this point, force a contraction, squeezing your abs, butt and the muscle between your legs. Hold this contraction for a couple of seconds.

variations

BASIC/INTERMEDIATE

Move the ball away from the wall so that it is less stabilized. You'll need to readjust your foot position on the ball so that you can raise your hips while preventing the ball from scooting out from under your feet.

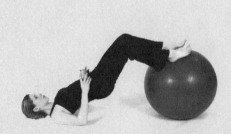

TIP

• You can press against the ground with your arms to help stabilize your body and to allow you to deepen the contraction.

• The benefit of the movement comes from holding the contraction, not from the amount of reps you perform.

2 Slowly lower your hips, but stop just short of allowing them to return to the starting position.

2

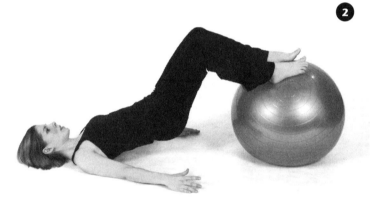

INTERMEDIATE/ADVANCED

Try performing this movement with only one foot on the ball at a time. Raise your other leg into the air and off to the side a bit to help counter-balance. Perform an equal number of reps with each foot off the ball.

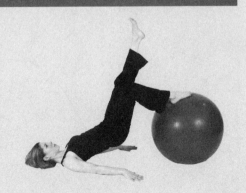

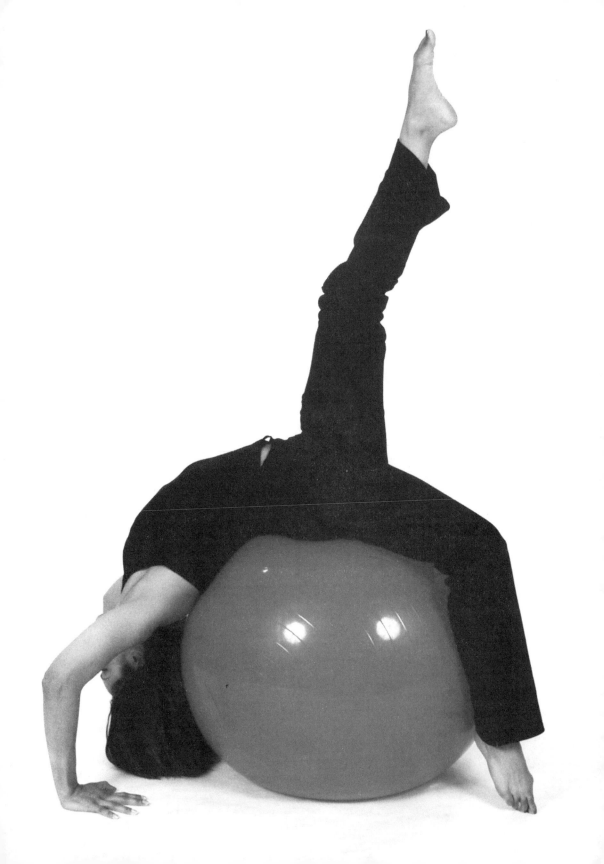

be flexible: stretches

One of the properties of the body most undertrained and neglected by many hardcore exercisers is flexibility. While building muscle mass or keeping your midsection toned are important for overall fitness, making certain that you can move through the entire range of motion that your body was intended is also critical for ideal fitness. Whatever level of fitness you are at, you should incorporate some or all of these movements in your day-to-day training. When you do, you'll find that not only do you move better, but you feel better and you're much less likely to suffer training-related or everyday injuries.

back bend stretch

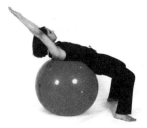

This can be a gentle or dynamic stretch to open up your back and lengthen your spine. The ball supports you, making it a safe way to stretch out a tight or injured back. It's also a good stretch for your abdominals.

STARTING POSITION: Lie with your back on the ball and your legs bent and your feet placed comfortably apart. Stretch your arms up overhead.

1 Stretch your arms farther, down toward the ground, reaching back as far as you can. You can shift the position of your feet to roll back a little farther and deepen the stretch.

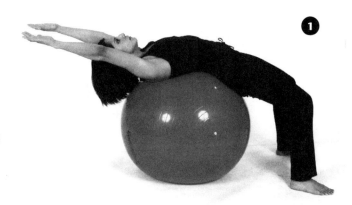

variations

INTERMEDIATE

If you are flexible enough, place your arms behind you on the ground to open your shoulders. In this position, contract the muscles of your middle back to further open your shoulders.

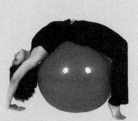

INTERMEDIATE/ADVANCED

Place your hands on the ground and lift your hips slightly up off the ball so that you are contacting it as little as possible, supporting as much of your weight as you can in the backbend position.

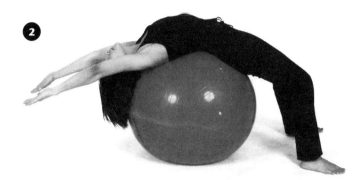

②

TIP

• You can also stretch your arms out to the side, arching your back left to right (as well as from your butt to your neck).

• Avoid pushing back too much because you may roll off the ball and hit your head. Not pretty.

2 Rock back and forth, as desired, and even side to side (but be careful not to lose your balance or put too much weight and pressure on one side).

3 Roll out of the position, back to the starting point, and then roll back into the position to deepen the stretch.

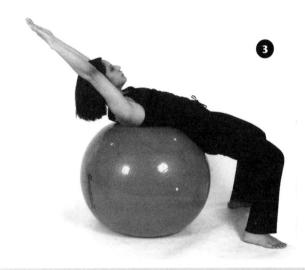

③

ADVANCED

Using some support from the ball, if needed, lift one leg as high as you can. Hold the position. Then repeat on the other side.

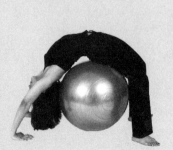

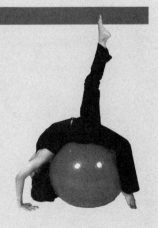

spine stretch

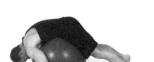

This position is the reverse of the back bend stretch since it takes your back through the opposite range of motion. It's great to pair these two stretches together (and throw in the side stretch, too!), allowing you to stretch your torso in all directions.

STARTING POSITION: Place your chest on the ball. Reach forward and stretch your arms out toward the ground. Position your feet about shoulder width apart. You should be on your toes with your legs bent a little.

1 Roll over the ball a little more by straightening your legs slightly, allowing the ball to travel forward. Roll back and bring your hands up onto the ball to increase the range of motion.

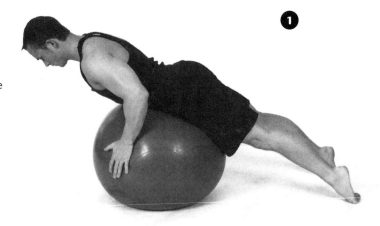

1

BASIC/INTERMEDIATE

Instead of placing your arms out in front of you, you can reach your arms out to the sides and place them on the ground, getting a good stretch in your shoulders and upper back.

variations

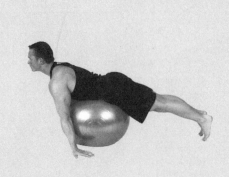

TIP

- Feel free to mix and match these various stretch positions, emphasizing the ones that feel good and the ones where you feel the tightest, but always keep your movements smooth. When you reach your deepest stretch position, hold it for several seconds. The objective is to elongate your body and enhance your flexibility.
- Take as much or as little time as you like stretching. You can stretch as a warm up, cool down, or short break between weight sets.

2 Lift your head and back, arching them up off the ball, looking up.

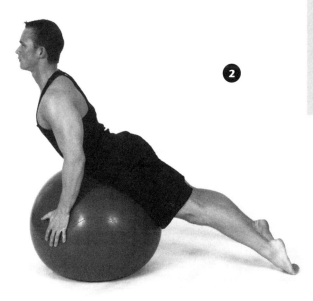

INTERMEDIATE/ADVANCED

With one hand on the ball and the ball under your abdomen and/or hips, twist to the side, extending one arm up as you arch your back. Twist back into position, placing that hand on the ball, and twist the other arm up and behind you.

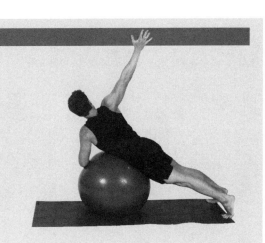

side stretch

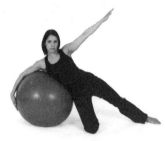

This stretch is a great way to open your body side to side, stretching out your obliques, abs and lats.

STARTING POSITION: Kneel alongside the ball. Reach out and grab the ball with one arm, and bring that side of your body in contact with the ball so that it supports your body weight. With the knee closest to the ball still on the ground, straighten the other leg and allow that foot to contact the ground for stability.

1

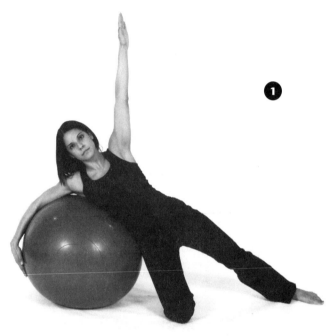

1 Stretch the arm that doesn't contact the ball up over your head.

variations

BASIC

For an easier stretch, you can perform this movement from a kneeling position beside the ball, rather than supported by the ball.

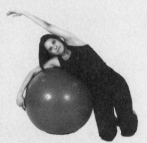

INTERMEDIATE

Place both feet on the ground with your legs straight, and only your side and arm in contact with the ball. This will move your point of stabilization much farther from the ball and increase the demands on both stabilization and flexibility.

2 Bend into the ball, taking your arm overhead and out toward parallel to the ground. You can allow the ball to roll under you just a little bit to help deepen the stretch, but maintain strict control over the ball's movement so that it doesn't scoot out from under you.

TIP

- Instead of extending your contact arm, you can place the forearm that touches the ball crosswise over the ball to help better stabilize your position.

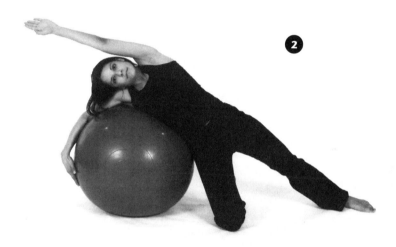

2

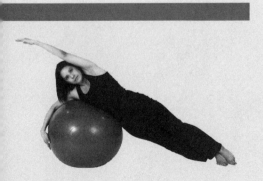

INTERMEDIATE/ADVANCED

With your knee closest to the ball on the ground, extend the other leg out straight, parallel and off ground.

hip stretch

The ball can be an excellent tool for helping you stretch out your lower body. This stretch and its variations are among the most crucial and basic types of lower-body stretches.

STARTING POSITION: Straddle the ball with one foot on the floor in front of you; the other leg should be behind you. Your legs can be slightly bent. Your feet should essentially be parallel even though they're far apart, with your toes pointing the same direction that you're facing. Place your hands on your hips or on the sides of the ball for stability.

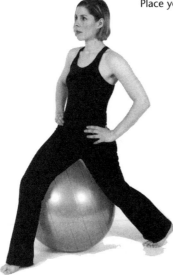

BASIC

Stretch your leg 90 degrees out to the side instead of behind you. This will stretch the muscles of your inner and outer thighs. Place your butt more against the front of the ball so that you are well supported and still able to get a good range of motion. Roll the ball away from your extended leg, deepening the stretch, but maintain your torso in its upright, neutral-spine position.

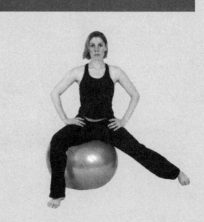

variations

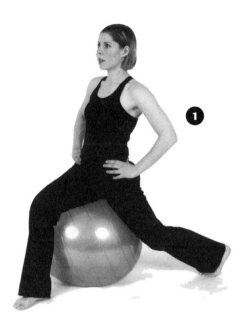

1

1 Inch your feet as far apart as is comfortable. You will feel a stretch in your hamstrings in your front leg, as well as a good stretch along the top of your trailing leg, in your quadriceps and hip flexors. Allow your body weight to sink into the ball to deepen the stretch. After a few seconds, try to move your feet a little farther apart: Switch leg positions and repeat.

INTERMEDIATE

Turn over your back foot so that the top of that foot is in contact with the ground. This will increase your stretch and separate your legs a little more. You can place your hands on your hips or extend your arms for balance.

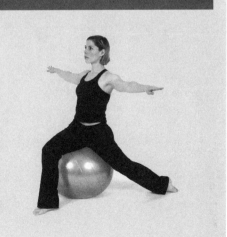

roll-out stretch

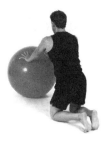

This is a great stretch for your upper body, particularly targeting your shoulder joints and the muscles of your back and shoulders. It's an excellent way to counter the stiffness in your neck, shoulders and back that comes from, for instance, sitting too long or working on a computer.

STARTING POSITION: Kneel in front of the ball and place your outstretched arms on the ball.

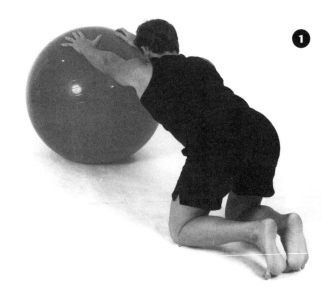

1

1 Roll the ball forward so that your upper body is close to parallel to the ground.

variations

INTERMEDIATE

With both arms on the ball and your knees on the ground, stretch across your body and feel a deep stretch on one side of your back. Twist your body the other way and stretch the other side as well.

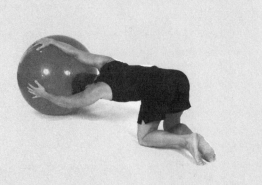

2 Using your hands and arms, roll the ball out farther away from your knees. Continue extending the ball—and your body—until you feel a good stretch in your shoulders and upper back.

TIP

- Hold the core of your body tight as you do this. This will help stabilize your body and help you keep control over your positioning and over the ball itself.

- Shift your body so that you settle back onto your heels. This will deepen the stretch in your back and shoulders. As you reach this stretch position, contract the muscles in the middle of your back.

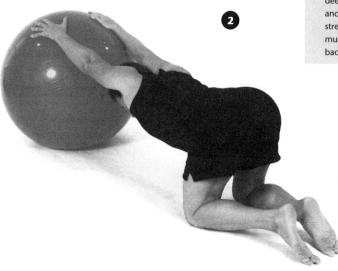

2

ADVANCED

To get a deeper stretch, angle your upper legs toward the ball so that your knees are farther away from it. You will have to support your body more with the ball. This can be a dynamic stretch so be sure to maintain body control at all times.

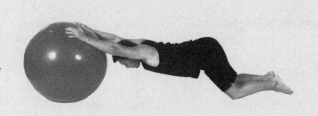

moving forward

After you've been training in a particular program for a few months, you may notice that your goals have begun to shift—as you shed body fat, you may find that you're more interested in toning up your body or adding more muscle mass. Or you may have the same goal, but you may recognize that you are not making progress at the same rate that you first did.

Both of these are good indicators that it's time to make modifications in your program. In fact, never forget that one of the best ways to continue to get great results from exercise is to regularly change your program. Eventually your body adapts to doing the same routine month after month, and you'll begin to plateau. Look for these points, and change your program by making one or more of the following substitutions:

CHANGE PROGRAMS: If your goal has begun to shift, it's time to move on to the program that addresses your new goal.

SUBSTITUTE EXERCISES: Even if your goal has not shifted, after three months of performing the same exercises, sets and reps, your body will be well accommodated to them. This book includes many different exercises for each of the various body parts. At this point, choose an exercise you have not been doing and substitute it for one that you have been doing for that same body part. For instance, you may substitute cross-body triceps extensions for triceps kickbacks. Or add hands on the ball push-ups in place of incline dumbbell presses.

ADD EXERCISES: Increase the volume of your training by simply adding more exercises instead of substituting.

MIX AND MATCH: Perform different exercises each time you work out instead of rigidly doing the same ones. For instance, try Planges (page 94), Pike Presses (page 112) or Shoulder Rotations (page 88) as substitute shoulder exercises. Regardless of your program, this will stimulate your body differently and better help you achieve your goals. Try a few exercises and see which ones you seem to like best and seem to give you the best results. I also like to include an exercise here or there that I don't like as much as others— sometimes the reason people don't like an exercise is that it addresses a weakness of the body. This can make it an important exercise to include.

CHANGE THE AMOUNT OF WEIGHT YOU USE: Experiment a little. Try a week where you use more weight (and fewer reps), then try another week where you use lighter weights (and higher reps). When you work your body in these different ways, you actually stimulate it considerably more than if you always just use the same weight. Lighter weights can really help you build muscular endurance while heavier weights help you build strength. If you're stronger and have more endurance, you are making yourself more fit overall.

INCREASE THE NUMBER OF SETS YOU PERFORM: In addition to adding exercises, you can add an extra set or two of your favorite exercises, or exercises that target a body part you want to focus on. Feel free to perform four or five sets of basic exercises such as wall squats or dumbbell presses instead of the two or three sets in your initial program.

SHORTEN REST PERIODS: This is an easy way to make your workouts tougher. Every once in awhile, try to shorten the amount of time you rest between sets of the same exercise. Try to do each set with only a minute of rest between sets. Then try it with only 30 seconds of rest. This challenges your muscles by giving them less time to recover.

muscle glossary

ABS: This term often refers to the rectus abdominis muscle (or the "six-pack" muscle), but it can refer more broadly to all the muscles in the abdominal region. Most abdominal exercises primarily target this dominant midsection muscle.

ABS, LOWER: These are simply the lower part of the rectus abdominis, or "abs."

ASSISTING MUSCLES: These are muscles that belong to a body part group other than the one you are targeting; for many exercises, it is impossible to target the primary muscle group without recruiting the assisting muscle group somewhat. For instance, triceps assist with many chest (pectoral) movements such as incline presses.

BICEPS: These muscles lie along the front of your upper arms.

BRACHIALIS: This arm muscle is positioned between the biceps and triceps, making only the edges visible through the skin. Look for it on the outer arm.

CALVES: These muscles run along the backs of the lower legs.

CORE: A generic term referring to all the muscles of the middle of the body, both front and back. These muscles include all those of the abdominals and lower back, as well as deeper muscles in these regions.

DELTOIDS (DELTS): These shoulder muscles consist of three major muscles, as well as several other stabilizing and smaller muscles. The *front delts* lie on the front of your shoulder, visible when you look at yourself straight on in the mirror. The *middle delts* are the dominant muscle of the shoulder group, lying along the outside of your shoulders, attaching to your upper arms. The *rear delts* are the smallest of the three delt heads, lying at the back of the shoulder where your shoulder joint meets your back.

GLUTES: The primary muscles of your butt.

HAMSTRINGS: This group of muscles runs from the backs of your knees to your hips.

HIP FLEXORS: These muscles attach your legs to your pelvis.

LATISSIMUS DORSI (LATS): The wide, flaring muscles of your mid- and upper back.

OBLIQUES: The finger-like muscles that lie alongside your abs.

PECTORALS (PECS): These chest muscles are a fairly simple muscle group responsible for pressing objects away from or bringing them across your body.

QUADRICEPS (QUADS): This major muscle group lies along the fronts of your upper thighs.

RHOMBOIDS: These small back muscles lie just above the lats and underneath your traps, just below your shoulder. Most exercises that target the lats also target the rhomboids, so, for the purposes of this book, the rhomboids do not need to be thought of as separate from the lats.

SPINAL ERECTORS: These lower back muscles are also part of your "core" but easily injured by performing exercises with poor form. Keeping your spine in its "neutral position" will help prevent injury to these (and other) muscles.

STABILIZER MUSCLES: The body is made up of over 600 muscles and, beyond the largest and most basic muscles, mentioning these muscles by name generally adds confusion rather than clarity. For this reason, I often call smaller muscles "stabilizers."

TRAPEZIUS (TRAPS): This muscle is shaped like a butterfly at the back of your neck and is not quite a back or shoulder muscle. The lower traps lie along your spine in your upper back, and the upper traps lie along the tops of your shoulders near your neck.

TRICEPS: Located along the backsides of the upper arms.

index

a

abdominal muscles 6
abdominal-strengthening exercises
138–55
abs crunches 140–43
cross-body twists 150–51
hip raises 154–55
reverse crunches 146–47
roll-up crunches 144–45
side crunches 148–49
side twists 152–153
abs crunches
back on ball 140–41
feet on ball 142–43
alternate biceps curls 50–51
ankle weights 9

b

back bend stretch 158–59
back extensions 120–21
reverse 122–23
back on ball exercises 66–81
abs crunches 140–41
back bend stretch 158–59
cross-body twists 150–51
flat chest flyes 72–73
flat chest presses 68–69
incline chest flyes 74–75
incline chest presses 70–71
incline curls 80–81
pullovers 76–77
triceps extensions 78–79
ball 8–9
benefits of 2, 5
choosing 8–9
biceps curls 50–51
blocks, for raises 10

body fat

body fat
reducing 3–4, 36
program 28–35

c

calf raises 136–37
cardio 15, 37
chest on ball exercises 82–97
dumbbell rows 96–97
front raises 86–87
plange 94–95
preacher curls 90–91
rear delt flyes 84–85
shoulder rotations 88–89
wrist curls 92–93
concentration curls 90–91
"core" 6
cross-body twists 150–51
crunches
abs crunches 140–43
reverse 146–47
roll-up 144–45
side 148–49

d

dumbbell rows
chest on ball 96–97
hands on ball 104–105

e

equipment 8–10
exercises 45–167
substituting 168

f

feet on ball exercises 108–17
abs crunches 142–43
hip raises 154–55

pikes presses 112–13
push-ups 110–11
triceps dips 116–17
walk-arounds 114–15
Firm Foundation program 20–27
flat chest flyes 72–73
flexibility 156–67
form 11–12
flat chest presses 68–69
front raises
chest on ball 86–87
seated 62–63

h

hammer curls 52–53
hamstrings curls 124–25
hand(s) on ball exercises 98–107
dumbbell rows 104–105
push-ups 100–101
triceps kickbacks 102–103
walk-arounds 106–107
hip raises 154–55
hip stretch 164–65

i

incline chest flyes 74–75
incline chest presses 70–71
incline curls 80–81
injury 6, 11, 13, 19, 40

l

lateral leg raises 134–35
lateral raises 58–59
leg strengtheners 118–37
back extensions 120–21
hamstrings curls 124–25
lateral leg raises 134–35
lunges 130–31

reverse back extensions 122–23
seated calf raises 136–37
side lunges 132–33
stiff-legged deadlifts 126–27
wall squats 128–29
lunges 130–31

m

mats 10
Muscle Bound program 36–43
muscles 3, 6–7
glossary 169

p

pikes presses 112–13
planges 94–95
posture 5
preacher curls 90–91
programs 18–43
changing 168
pullovers 76–77
push-ups
feet on ball 110–11
hands on ball 100–101
pyramiding
defined 14

r

rear delt flyes 84–85
recovery time 7
reps 11–12, 15, 37
reverse back extensions 122–23
reverse crunches 146–47
roll-up crunches 144–45
roll-out stretch 166–67

s

seated calf raises 136–37

seated exercises 48–65
alternate biceps curls 50–51
front raises 62–63
hammer curls 52–53
lateral raises 58–59
shoulder presses 60–61
shrugs 64–65
side twists 152–53
triceps extensions 54–55
triceps kickbacks 56–57
shoulder presses 60–61
shoulder rotations 88–89
shrugs 64–65
side crunches 148–49
side lunges 132–33
side stretch 162–63
side twists 152–53
Slim and Trim program 28–35
spine stretch 160–61
stiff-legged deadlifts 126–27
stretches 156–67
back bend stretch 158–59
hip stretch 164–65
roll-out stretch 166–67
side stretch 162–63
spine stretch 160–61
stretching 13–14
exercises 156–67
toning
defined 20
program 20–27

t

triceps dips 116–17
triceps extensions
back on ball 78–79
seated 54–55
triceps kickbacks

hand on ball 102–103
seated 56–57

w

walk-arounds
feet on ball 114–15
hands on ball 106–107
wall 10
wall squat curls 128
wall squats 128–29
warming up 13–14, 37
weight bench 9
weight levels 19
changing 168
weights
benefits of 2, 3–4
choosing 9
wrist curls
palm down 93
palm up 92

about the author

STEVEN STIEFEL, the author of *Fit in 15*, has been a health and fitness writer for over a decade and is currently the nutrition editor at *FLEX Magazine*. Previously, he was a contributing editor at *Men's Fitness* magazine. He also writes articles for *Muscle & Fitness*, *HERS* and other health and fitness publications. Steven earned his master's degrees at the University of Arizona and the University of Southern California. His short fiction has appeared in *The Georgia Review*, *McSweeney's* and other publications. In addition to his writing career, Steven also serves as Chief Creative Officer for Ronick Productions (www.ronickproductions.com), a feature film company located in Los Angeles.

other books by ulysses press

FIT IN 15: 15-MINUTE MORNING WORKOUTS THAT BALANCE CARDIO, STRENGTH, AND FLEXIBILITY
Steven Stiefel, $14.95
Fit in 15 details a unique, full-body fitness program that even the busiest person can work into a morning schedule. The fun and flexible "7 days/7 workouts" plan lets readers choose from 55 specially designed 15-minute workouts.

ULTIMATE CORE BALL WORKOUT: STRENGTHENING AND SCULPTING EXERCISES WITH OVER 200 STEP-BY-STEP PHOTOS
Jeanine Detz, $14.95
Maximizes core training by tapping the power of the exercise ball with these strengthening and sculpting exercises.

THE GOLFER'S GUIDE TO PILATES: STEP-BY-STEP EXERCISES TO STRENGTHEN YOUR GAME
Monica Clyde, $14.95
Uses Pilates' combination of strength, flexibility, balance and mental focus to lower your score and improve every aspect of the game.

ELLIE HERMAN'S PILATES MATWORK PROPS WORKBOOK: STEP-BY-STEP GUIDE WITH OVER 200 PHOTOS
Ellie Herman, $12.95
Explains how props can enhance Pilates: the magic circles tone arms, the small ball held between the legs shapes thighs, the foam roller stretches the chest and shoulders, and the large exercise ball builds core stability.

To order these books call 800-377-2542 or 510-601-8301, fax 510-601-8307, e-mail ulysses@ulyssespress.com, or write to Ulysses Press, P.O. Box 3440, Berkeley, CA 94703. All retail orders are shipped free of charge. California residents must include sales tax. Allow two to three weeks for delivery.